EATING on the RUN

Second Edition

Evelyn Tribole, MS, RD

Leisure Press
Champaign, Illinois

Library of Congress Cataloging-in-Publication Data

Tribole, Evelyn, 1959-
    Eating on the run / Evelyn Tribole.--2nd ed.
    p. cm.
    Includes bibliographical references and index.
    ISBN 0-88011-452-5 (soft cover)
    1. Nutrition.   2. Time management.   I. Title.
    RA784.T75   1992
    613.2--dc20   91-19917
                                                         CIP

ISBN: 0-88011-452-5

Acquisitions Editor: Brian Holding; **Developmental Editor:** Lori Garrett; **Assistant Editors:** Laura Bofinger, Elizabeth Bridgett, Valerie Hall, Dawn Levy, and Kari Nelson; **Copyeditor:** Jane Bowers; **Proofreader:** Dawn Levy; **Indexer:** Barbara Cohen; **Production Director:** Ernie Noa; **Typesetters:** Angela K. Snyder and Kathy Fuoss; **Text Design:** Keith Blomberg; **Text Layout:** Tara Welsch and Angela K. Snyder; **Cover Design:** Jack Davis; **Cover Photo:** Lori Garrett; **Printer:** Versa Press

Leisure Press books are available at special discounts for bulk purchase for sales promotions, premiums, fund-raising, or educational use. Special editions or book excerpts can also be created to specification. For details, contact the Special Sales Manager at Leisure Press.

Printed in the United States of America   10 9 8 7 6 5

Leisure Press
A Division of Human Kinetics
P.O. Box 5076, Champaign, IL 61825-5076
1-800-747-4457

Canada: Human Kinetics, Box 24040, Windsor, ON N8Y 4Y9
1-800-465-7301 (in Canada only)

Europe: Human Kinetics, P.O. Box IW14, Leeds LS16 6TR, England
0532-781708

Australia: Human Kinetics, P.O. Box 80, Kingswood 5062, South Australia
618-374-0433

New Zealand: Human Kinetics, P.O. Box 105-231, Auckland 1
(09) 309-2259

To Krystin—you have enriched my life by dimensions I never knew existed and have given me a new perspective of what it means to be eating on the run.

Contents

Lists

Tables

Foreword

I was delighted when I was asked to write this foreword, because it was 4 years ago, through *Eating On the Run*'s first edition, that I met Evelyn Tribole. I was impressed by the book's thoroughness of information, simplicity of style, and energy of delivery! I immediately had to call Evelyn and tell her so.

Four years later, this new edition retains all the best of the first, but it is tailor-made to make eating well in the fast-paced '90s not only possible, but FUN! Evelyn's strategy of "progress, not perfection," and the concept of "no forbidden foods" are in step with the '90s approach to health. A focus on wellness is reflected in Evelyn's emphasis on building a healthy diet every day, rather than eliminating foods from your diet. It's a positive and reassuring approach to eating well that teaches you that highly nutritious choices abound wherever you go, whether to a deli, coffee shop, fast-food restaurant, or airline diner high in the skies. You'll learn to head off the hungries at the pass by adopting a few simple planning strategies for deciding when and what to eat even while in your car or at your desk.

I lovingly refer to Evelyn as *Shape*'s nutrition doctor, and now she can become yours. She's like the classical physician who works hard to keep you well, but most significantly gives you the tools you'll need so you can be your own nutrition doctor.

Dive into this book. Its combination of recipes, strategies, basic knowledge, and tips contain all the fundamentals to making nutrition work for you, regardless of your lifestyle. Make this book your stepping stone to a whole new way of living and thinking that leads to a healthier and higher quality of life. And as you begin, think about the fact that you're not giving up anything. Rather, you're getting the gift of health which nobody can give to you but yourself. After all, you're worth it!

Barbara Harris
Editor
Shape

Preface

Time is likely to be the scarcest and most coveted commodity in the '90s, according to a recent cover story in *Time* magazine.

Many activities compete with eating for time in our fragmented schedules. Skipping breakfast to catch an early morning meeting and running errands during lunch are examples of how the time famine is managed. Revolving dinner schedules are replacing family meals as more and more women work outside the home and everyone is on the run. All of these factors are moving us away from traditional meals.

In a 1990 Gallup poll, 64% of the people surveyed combined eating with another activity such as working, reading, or watching television. Almost 50% of the people stated that on a typical night they relied on frozen, packaged, or take-out meals for dinner.

I have seen these new trends emerging in my family, as well as with my patients, so I know how these trends can adversely affect eating and health. That is why *Eating on the Run* was completely revised and updated. The new edition is packed with more information and yet is still easy to read. I've added 9 new chapters, 30 new tables, and 2 new appendixes.

For those who are falling victim to occupational eating hazards such as long work hours, there's a whole new chapter devoted to this problem. It offers lots of easy tips to manage food in and around the workplace.

If you've found time to visit the grocery store lately, you probably were bombarded with over 26,000 foods to choose from, of which over half have no nutritional information on the food labels. A special chapter on the worst and best convenience foods found in a grocery store will help you find a streamlined solution to the shopping dilemma.

The growing proliferation of frozen meals demands a chapter of its own. Even the innocent-sounding "light" 300-calorie meals can camouflage fat traps and salt mines. Best bets in these categories are highlighted for easy selection. And for quick reference, a new appendix lists nutritional data for light frozen foods.

Of course, the food-service industry has responded to our time crunch by offering a variety of services and menu items. The chapters about fast foods and restaurants have been completely revised and updated, and now include best bets for eating out, and a new appendix provides nutritional information about fast-food menu items. Chapters on delis and airline meals have been added so that you'll know how to eat nutritiously no matter where you are.

And because most of us are not at home when a snack attack strikes, a new chapter contains suggestions for satisfying a sweet tooth whenever and wherever the urge happens.

It's no surprise to find that if Mom and Dad are eating on the run, so are their kids. That's why a new chapter has been devoted to the special issue of children on the run.

For those times that you just want to "eat on automatic pilot," chapter 20 contains a one-week eating plan that requires *no* cooking. This plan is uniquely flexible for a busy schedule.

The new *Eating on the Run* is a survival tool and a resource handbook, packed with easy-to-find information to get you through the '90s and beyond.

Acknowledgments

Sincere thanks and appreciation to the following people for their help and support:

- JoAnn Hattner, MPH, RD, of Stanford University Medical Center for her technical review of chapter 15, ''Kids on the Run''
- Bettye Nowlin, MPH, RD, Mary Farrell, and Elaine Roberts for review and comments
- Lori Garrett, my developmental editor, for her patience and support
- The food companies that shared their nutrition data
- All my clients and patients, who have taught me the realistic side of nutrition
- Most of all my husband, Jeff—my personal editor and official recipe timer (his coaching experience makes him a natural with a stopwatch). Little did he know that for better or worse really meant for better or *busy*.

1

Nutrition in a Nutshell

"I am lucky to eat breakfast before I go to sleep at night."—

overworked client

Sometimes we are so busy trying to "have it all" that we postpone essential things—like eating. Lunch-skipping has increased by 65% over the past decade. And many have fallen into the habit of waiting to eat until they get home and then eating one large meal.

If we're too busy to eat, when will we find time to cook or shop for groceries?

Feeling overwhelmed? You're not alone. Busy lifestyles do influence how and what we eat. Consider these trends:

200 fast-food hamburgers are eaten each second.

Americans consume one third of their calories eating out.

A 1990 Gallup poll revealed these meal trends:

- 50% of adults rely on frozen, packaged, or take-out meals for dinner.
- Over one third of adults said they rarely have more than 30 minutes to fix a meal.

- One out of four adults said that speed and ease of preparation are the most important factors when buying food.

In my counseling practice, I've noticed that fewer people are actually cooking. It's more like assembling a meal, if even that. My patients often are embarrassed to admit that they seldom cook or that they don't even—gasp—like cooking.

Don't apologize. You are busy. End of story. But does being busy have to mean poor nutrition and bad eating habits? Not at all.

Yet many people feel that if they can't eat perfectly, they are better off just ignoring the whole issue—waiting until they really will have the time . . . some day. Wrong. Wrong. Wrong. This perfectionist thinking trap can lead to a downward spiral of problems.

One bad food, one bad meal, or one off day of eating will not make or break you nutritionally. It's what you eat on a consistent basis that counts. Here are some other prevailing myths that could lead you into a nutritional inferiority complex:

Myth 1. You need to have three square meals for optimal nutrition.
Myth 2. If meals are not cooked or hot, they are inferior, especially lunch and dinner.
Myth 3. Snacking is unhealthy and leads to weight gain.
Myth 4. If you eat out often, rely on frozen meals, and eat fast food, you are doomed to poor health.
Myth 5. Eating healthy takes a lot of time.

If you are making hasty food choices because your stomach is desperate—which at the time means anything looks good and who cares about cholesterol, fat, and so forth—you could be cultivating future health problems.

Poor eating habits are like cigarette smoking: Their ill effects may not become evident for many years, but they can damage your health. You can eat a high-cholesterol diet for a long time without feeling your arteries slamming shut. Consequently, many people put off seeking good nutrition until their health is compromised. Ironically, the benefits of healthy eating are usually noticed rather quickly, usually in terms of more energy. (This is especially the case for meal skippers.)

Now is the time to get started. Aim for progress not perfection. First, get an idea of where your weaknesses are.

To begin, let's take a quick look at how your lifestyle affects your eating. Then you'll do a painless nutrition audit, and I'll give some simple nutrition tips to help save you from the hazards of fast-track eating. The subsequent chapters will focus on specific problem areas such as fast foods, frozen meals, and traveling.

By the way, if you are too busy to read this book, turn straight to chapter 20 for automatic pilot eating. It will serve as a Band-Aid approach to healthy eating on the run.

LIFESTYLE QUIZ

Size up your eating on the run lifestyle by taking this short quiz. Answer yes or no to the following questions:

1. Would you rather hit the snooze alarm than eat breakfast?
2. Are you too tired to cook at the end of the day?
3. Would you rather run errands or get extra work done than eat lunch?
4. Do you eat out often (this includes fast food and takeout)?
5. Are your cupboards and refrigerator often bare because you have trouble getting to the grocery store?
6. Do you find yourself playing vending machine roulette in the afternoons to suppress hunger pangs (most often choosing between a candy bar and chips)?
7. When eating out do you clean your plate?
8. Do you ever skip meals or go longer than 5 hours without eating?
9. Do you travel frequently?
10. Do you suffer from ''eating amnesia,'' that is, you can't remember what you ate or nibbled on during the course of a day?
11. Do you hate cooking? (Be honest with yourself.)
12. Do you rely on coffee to jump-start your brain throughout the day?
13. To save time, do you wait until the end of the day to eat one large meal?
14. Do you work 45 or more hours per week or combine two or more of the following responsibilities: job; school; child rearing; or active membership in a professional, charitable, or social organization? Or do you just always feel too busy?
15. Do you wait until the last moment to decide what to eat and then fall prey to your environment or mood?

A yes response to any of these questions could be a significant trouble spot. Add your yes responses to see how your eating lifestyle rates:

- 10-15: Eating gets in the way of your day. You are probably too busy to think about getting sick. You need to maximize your limited eating times.

- 5-9: You could be developing poor eating patterns; now is the time to make some changes.
- 1-4: Not bad, but you probably need to work on consistency.

NUTRITION AUDIT

To see how well you are feeding yourself, take this quick nutrition audit. Do you do the following?

- Eat a minimum of 5 servings from a combination of fruits and vegetables daily
- Eat at least 6 grain servings (cereals, breads, pasta, rice, and so forth) daily
- Consume two or more nonfat or lowfat dairy products daily
- Eat a maximum of 7 ounces of meat a day
- Eat beans regularly, at least three times a week
- Drink at least 8 cups (64 ounces) of water daily
- Eat a wide variety of foods (or is it always the same thing for breakfast, lunch, and dinner?)
- Eat sweets (cakes, cookies, doughnuts, pastries, ice cream, candy) often
- Eat fatty foods (chips, fries, dressings, large meat servings, sandwiches "heavy on the mayo") often
- Eat salty foods (soups, pickles, frozen meals, packaged or canned foods) often

How you rate: For the first 7 items, the answer should be yes. For the final three items, the answer should be no. If your answers "deviated" from the correct responses, you might be headed for nutritional distress.

Don't worry if the lifestyle and nutritional self-assessments reveal that you have many trouble spots. I will show you how to eat healthy no matter how frenetic your schedule is. But first, a word of warning about an often-tried method that doesn't work.

As I'll discuss in chapter 14, you cannot solve your nutritional problems simply by swallowing vitamin pills. Nutritional problems in the United States more often are caused by excesses (especially of fat) than by deficiencies.

NUTRITION BOOTCAMP: JUST THE BASICS

Obviously you're busy, so I will present the nutrition basics in a nutshell—just enough to get you by for now.

Nutrition Scorecard

One of the easiest ways to keep track of your nutrition is through a food grouping system. Surely, you are familiar with the Basic Four food groups. Dull and boring, right? Even though it seems like "ancient" nutrition, most people do not know how to use this simple system.

A 1990 Gallup poll sponsored in part by the American Dietetic Association revealed that although 78% of surveyed adults said they were familiar with the Basic Four, only 22% could actually name the groups. Imagine if they were asked to cite the servings!

The landmark 1989 *Diet and Health Report* by the National Research Council has led to some new food group adjustments. More servings of grains and fruits and vegetables are recommended for optimal health.

In April 1990, the California Department of Health Services took this report one step further and recommended the addition of legumes (beans) at least three times a week. The nutritional potency of beans is incredible, and for optimal health, it makes sense to include them regularly. (For more information on beans, see chapter 22.)

Nutrition Countdown

Here's an easy way to integrate the food grouping system and make it work for you.

6 (6 servings of grains)
5 (5 servings of fruits and vegetables)
4 (4 to 7 ounces of lean meats or alternatives)
3 (3 servings of beans *per week*)
2 (2 lowfat or nonfat dairy servings for men, and 3 for women)

To help remember the order of food groups and to count down toward good nutrition, remember this little mnemonic device:

"Good	food	maximizes	benefits	daily"
r	r	e	e	a
a	u	a	a	i
i	i	t	n	r
n	t/	s/	s	y
s	v	a		
	e	l		
	g	t		
	s.	s.		

Here are examples and serving sizes for each food group:

Grains. 1/2 cup of rice, pasta, or cereal; or one slice of bread. (Note: Focus on choosing whole grains where possible.)

Fruits and Vegetables. 1/2 cup or one piece. Include green and yellow vegetables, and citrus fruits.

Meats and Meat Alternatives. 4 to 7 ounces. Choose lean meat, poultry, or fish. (Beans can also be included here.) Limit eggs to four per week (1 egg = 1 ounce). Here's a gauge to eyeball your meat consumption without measuring:

1 chicken breast (skinless)	=	3-5 ounces
1 chicken thigh (skinless)	=	2-3 ounces
1 egg	=	1 ounce
1 lean hamburger patty	=	3 ounces
1 lean steak	=	6 ounces or more

Beans. Three times weekly: 1/2 cup dried beans cooked or 3/4 cup bean soup. Remember that beans can count as a meat serving because they are rich in protein.

Dairy. 1 cup yogurt or milk, or 1-1/2 ounces lowfat cheese. Quality counts, so choose nonfat and lowfat forms.

Variety

Of course, variety is important. You know that. But how often do you get stuck eating the same old thing for breakfast or eating at the same restaurant for lunch and ordering ''the usual''? Certainly this is an easy way to eat; it requires no thinking. But the downside is, not only can this be boring, but you might be placing yourself in a nutritional rut.

Variety is important not only to ensure you get the 50-some nutrients that you need. It also distributes any possible risks (environmental contaminants, for example) that might be in the food you eat.

Try simple changes for variety. For example, vary the type of cereals, mix them, even rotate brands. Change the type of juice you drink. With so many different real fruit juices and blends to choose from, there's no excuse to settle on just one.

Balance

Just remember the 6-5-4-3-2 Nutrition Countdown.

Moderation

This is such a worn-out goal of nutritious eating that ev
Thesaurus gives as an example of moderation, "was advised ... .
drink with moderation." Moderation is an admirable goal without
direction. I feel that its dictum is anemic when trying to change eating
habits. I am throwing moderation to the wind—I will give you specific
examples and tools throughout this book of how to use moderation
in your eating habits.

OTHER KEYS: FINDING TIME TO EAT

One food industry executive predicted that the two most important
timesaving devices for eating will be the fax machine and the car!

If you have just 60 seconds, you have time to eat nutritiously! Remember, there is no nutrition commandment etched in stone man-
dating that you sit down to a big meal. Tight schedules call for tight
eating, which can easily be achieved through a form of snacking
known as grazing. I am going to show you quick and easy ways to
get good nutrition in one minute or less, regardless of your schedule.
Of course, a little bit of planning will be essential (but still easy).

THREE EASY GUIDELINES TO REMEMBER

1. Countdown to nutrition using 6-5-4-3-2.
2. Go no longer than 5 hours without eating. Why 5 hours? Your
   body's primary energy source is glucose. Glucose is stored in
   the liver as glycogen and normally runs out in 4 to 6 hours. If
   you do not re-fuel the liver glycogen with food (carbohydrates),
   your body will be running on empty and will have to resort
   to "creative fueling." This can particularly affect brainpower
   because your brain uses glucose exclusively for energy.
3. Choose primarily foods that have no more than 3 grams of fat
   for every 100 calories. This will keep your fat level within the
   goal of less than 30% fat calories a day.

2

Grazing for Survival

"I have no time to eat, so I just drink coffee all day long until I get home."—

television news reporter

Even if you only have time to gulp down a cup of coffee, you still can graze your way to good nutrition. (There's hope—don't throw in the towel.) In this chapter, you'll learn about grazing, a simple way to bring nutrition into your on-the-run lifestyle.

TIMESAVING TRAP: SKIPPING MEALS

Let's look at the problems with skipping meals or going so long without eating that it's like minifasting.

Skip Now, and Pay Later

As the mechanic in the Fram oil filter commercial says, "You can pay me now, or pay me later," meaning that investing in a high quality

filter will alleviate costly future repairs. Similarly, investing in a he
snack or quick meal can help you avoid costly nutrition mistakes
example, skipping breakfast, or any meal for that matter, will catch up
with you. Your body eventually gets overly hungry later on in the day.
Let's face it: When you are famished, anything goes. All honorable
intentions fly out the window.

Consider these other consequences of meal skipping:

- People who skip meals, especially breakfast, tend to have lower
  metabolism rates. When metabolism is lowered, it's more difficult to lose weight.
- Nearly 90% of dieters skip meals.
- According to the American Dietetic Association, a person who
  eats breakfast tends to burn more calories at that time, as well as
  throughout the day.
- Meal skippers don't perform as well: They accomplish less work,
  are physically less steady, and are slower making decisions.
- Brain fuel, glucose, is compromised within 4 to 6 hours if you have
  not eaten. Glucose, stored in the liver as glycogen, runs out during
  this time period. The liver is like the traffic cop for blood sugar.
  When blood glucose dips too low, the liver releases glucose (from
  the glycogen) into the blood. But if the glycogen is gone, the body
  has to turn to "creative fueling" that is less efficient.
- Calorie loading occurs if you eat most of the day's energy needs
  in one meal, usually dinner. Eating a large meal, even though
  it's just one meal, tends to overwhelm your body with calories
  that it does not need at that moment. And you know where the
  body puts the extra calories it doesn't need—in fat on the waist,
  hips, thighs, and so forth.

Overcoming the Skipping Rut

Despite the side effects of meal skipping, it's easy to get caught in
the trap of doing without. Here are a few scenarios to show how
easily this occurs:

Breakfast:	Got up too late; never hungry; nothing to eat
Lunch:	Tied up in meetings; running errands; forgot to bring lunch; not enough cash
Dinner:	After-work meeting; evening aerobics class; arrive home "too late"

Okay, okay. Maybe you are not hungry in the morning. "Can't eat,"
you say. You probably have conditioned your body over a number of
years not to be hungry.

And who has time to eat, really? Dilemma.

Remember, you don't need to sit down to three big meals. Instead you can try fast, nutritious mini-meals, especially when time is short. For example, breakfast is just a matter of having *something* to eat in the morning, even if you have to wait until you get to the office. The ultimate quick minibreakfast could be as easy as a glass of juice and a glass of milk—it takes all of 19 seconds to prepare. Enter grazing.

GRAZING

Grazing is simply eating small mini-meals or snacks throughout the day. You can eat whenever or wherever you want—at home or on the job, at any time of the day. This flexibility should fit anyone's schedule. With grazing, you are only a bite away from your next meal.

Graze Craze

It is quite clear that grazing is not a fad but a trend that is here to stay. The *Wall Street Journal* documented the trend in 1988 with a feature story headlined, ''Are Square Meals Headed for Extinction?'' Aptly, the illustration showed a graveyard with headstones inscribed ''breakfast,'' ''lunch,'' and ''dinner.''

In 1989, the U.S. Department of Agriculture (USDA) also recognized the grazing trend. A spokesperson for the USDA acknowledged in an official news release that grazing or snacking can be a healthy way of eating: ''It's not how you eat, but *what* you eat.''

Extra Benefits

There are many advantages to grazing. It is one of the most convenient ways to eat, and it is workable regardless of your schedule.

Besides the timesaving benefit, many studies demonstrate the nutritional merits of grazing. Scientifically, these are often referred to as ''nibbling versus gorging'' studies.

Lower Cholesterol

A promising study reported in the *New England Journal of Medicine* in 1990 demonstrated that a grazing diet resulted in lower serum cholesterol. Subjects were divided into two different groups and given identical diets. The only difference was how they ate. One group was given a "nibbling" diet which consisted of 17 snacks a day! The other group had their food divided into three meals. The researchers concluded that a nibbling diet, or increased meal frequency, could play a role in the prevention of heart disease. (I'm not suggesting that you have to eat 17 times daily. This was an extreme eating pattern.)

Brainpower

To illustrate the brainpower of timely snacking or grazing, let's consider the results of this 1990 study by Kanarek and Swinney. Subjects given fruited yogurt for an afternoon snack had a significant increase in mental performance compared to those who had only a diet soda. (The researchers measured mental performance by giving a battery of tests that included memory tests, math reasoning, reading, and attention span.)

Think about how often you might try to tide yourself over with a diet beverage or a cup of coffee. You may be temporarily fooling your stomach, but it catches up with you.

Weight Control

Snacking can help manage weight. Ironically, despite the metabolic benefits of grazing, many people think of snacking as a no-no. They fear that it may lead to gaining weight, when it can do just the opposite.

More often than not, when I ask clients at what time do they experience hunger or feel most vulnerable to eating, they reply "in the afternoon." Next, I ask what they do about this urge. The typical reply is "nothing," they ride it out.

Frequently, I have seen people play "meal martyr" by going 8 hours or longer until their next meal. For example, if you have lunch, say at noon, but you work late and don't get home until 8 p.m.—your body is running on empty.

As a consequence, by the time you get home from work or have an opportunity to eat, you are more likely to gorge.

A small healthy snack such as lowfat crackers with lowfat cheese will take the edge off hunger. This is especially useful to do before going out to eat or out to a party—it helps promote more controlled eating. See List 2.1 for some snack ideas for calorie counters.

List 2.1
Snacks for the Calorie Conscious

These foods are lower in sugar and fat than other more traditional snack foods. Remember, eating these should be a conscious activity. Enjoy!

Corn tortilla
Diet gelatin
Fresh fruit
   Apple
   Banana
   Grapefruit
   Grapes
   Melon
   Peach
   Pineapple
   Orange
Frozen plain banana
Graham crackers
100% juice bar
Low- or nonfat cottage cheese
Lowfat crackers
   Ak-mak
   Finn Crisp
   Kavli Flatbread
   Melba toast

Pogens Krisprolls
RyKrisp
Wasa
Matzo crackers
Minibagels
Minibox of raisins
Nonfat milk
Nonfat yogurt
Raw vegetables
   Broccoli
   Carrot sticks
   Cauliflower
   Celery stalks
   Cherry tomatoes
   Mushrooms
Rice cakes
Toast
Tofu
Vanilla wafers
Vegetable soup

WHAT TYPE OF GRAZER ARE YOU?

A market research survey by Campbell Food Service divided grazers into the following five categories:

Sheepish Grazers.   Most of their grazing is done at home. They enjoy small simple foods such as nuts, fruits, and cheese.

Convenient Grazers.   They snack at convenience stores or drive-through restaurants. Convenient Grazers are nomadic eaters who do no planning or shopping.

Lone Grazers.   Food just gets in their way, but they do not allow it to interfere with other activities. They are apt to engage in "paired eating" (eating while doing something else, such as working, reading, or driving).

World-Class Grazers.   These individuals like sophistication and variety in their foods. They prefer delicacies such as Brie cheese and filled croissants.

Freudian Grazers.   They eat to relieve emotional hunger, such as stress or boredom. Freudian Grazers like sweets or spicy foods with good texture.

Of these grazing personas, I consider the Convenient Grazer and the Freudian Grazer styles potentially hazardous to your health.

Because Convenient Grazers do no planning, their nutritional intake is haphazard and likely to be high in fat. If you fall into this category, don't be alarmed. The following chapters will show you how to plan successfully, without a lot of hassle, for eating on the run.

Freudian Grazers tend to drown their emotions in food. Emotional hunger will not be satisfied by food. Eating is only a means of temporary relief that is very short lived. This negative habit can lend itself to compulsive overeating and obesity. Strategies for coping with emotional eating are discussed in chapter 12.

If you tend to be a Freudian Grazer and eat for relief, start asking yourself, "Why am I eating?" The only good answer to that question is, "Because I am hungry."

PITFALLS OF GRAZING

To improve your snacking or grazing, you should be aware of other possible problems that can occur.

Eating Amnesia

This syndrome occurs with mindless eating. You forget what (or more likely, how much) you have eaten. Most people have trouble remembering what they ate for their last meal, let alone a "bite of this, and a spoonful of that."

Nibblers start out innocently with little tasters here and there. The next thing you know, a whole box of crackers or bag of cookies is gone—and you were the only person around that day. You may swear that a ravenous ghost lives in your kitchen, but take a close look in the mirror and you'll see who the culprit is.

To avoid becoming a victim of eating amnesia, try these approaches to becoming a conscious eater:

1. Have your snacks predetermined, such as five crackers and lowfat cheese, and put them in a baggie or bowl. You can nibble on them throughout the day, but when the bowl is empty, you will know that you indeed ate five crackers.
2. Keep a mental record of what you are eating and compare it to the 6-5-4-3-2 Nutrition Countdown system.

Stress Breakers and Emotional Relief

Because we are so busy, most people do not feel comfortable about taking a deserved break and doing "nothing." Most people I counsel would never sit at a desk for their break because "it would look lazy." But it's okay to eat—eating looks productive. Consequently, to get a break, many people turn to food, even when they are not hungry. Food becomes the acceptable time-out.

Advertising

Many food companies exploit any iota of nutrition to make their foods sound redeeming (such as potato chips dusted with oat bran). Healthy-sounding food labels may give the illusion of wholesomeness, even when the opposite is true. Here are some examples to watch out for:

Healthy-sounding	*But . . .*
Fruit rolls/bits	Often high in sugar
Granola bars	Often loaded with fat and sugar
Juice drinks	Contain little juice
Microwave popcorn	Often high in fat
No-cholesterol chips	High in fat

And beware of the commercial traps that lure you into believing that a candy bar (or equivalent) is a nutritious treat to carry you over. Candy bars are usually packed with fat and sugar.

RULES FOR SUCCESSFUL GRAZING

To enjoy the benefits of grazing, here are some guidelines to keep you on the right course to quick, healthy eating:

1. *Go no longer than 5 hours without eating.* If you wait any longer, you are more likely to get into trouble. If you normally go hours

without eating, try this little test. Record your energy level throughout the day. You will probably notice your low or tired times correspond to long stretches between eating.

2. *Choose foods from the 6-5-4-3-2 Nutrition Countdown system.* Grazing foods should fulfill at least one of the food group servings. This will assure you get adequate nutrition from your snack. You may want to simply keep a running total in your head. Or you can keep track with the following slash-tally method:

Grains	Fruits/Vegs.	Meats/Alts.	Beans	Dairy
~~IIII~~ I	~~IIII~~	IIII	III	II

You can track this on a Post-It note kept in your appointment book or wherever is convenient.

3. *Choose nutrient-dense foods.* This means choosing foods that have the most nutrition for the mouthful in the least amount of calories. Caution: Many processed snack foods, such as chips, candy, and some granola bars are loaded with fat and sugar. For example, advertisements tell how a Snickers candy bar can "satisfy" you, but the nutritional price is costly: 510 calories and 24 grams of fat in a king-size bar. Yikes!

4. *Foods need to be portable and ready-to-go.* Think how often you have made noble attempts to graze on vegetables, only to find them buried at the bottom of your refrigerator, wilted. Solution: They should be washed and ready to grab.

5. *The food item needs to be accessible.* If you're working through lunch, your snacks need to be stashed in a briefcase or desk drawer. List 2.2 offers some handy ideas for snacks to stash.

List 2.2
Snacks for the Briefcase or Desk Drawer

The following snacks are especially handy to have for those days when you are racing against the clock. The foods listed here travel well.

Bagel	Half sandwich
Bran muffin	Juice (paper cartons)
Bread sticks	Lowfat crackers
Dried fruit	Lowfat cheese and crackers
Apples	Raisin bread
Apricots	Raw vegetables
Peaches	Rice cakes
Pears	Snack-sized canned tuna
Raisins	Unsweetened cereal
Fig bars	Whole wheat roll
Fresh fruit	

Perhaps you are fortunate and your place of employment has a refrigerator. Take advantage of it! Your options are greatly increased when refrigeration is possible. List 2.3 provides you with some possibilities. Or, if you don't have access to a refrigerator or are on the road a lot, you might consider using a portable cooler. Also see chapter 11, ''Occupational Eating Hazards.''

List 2.3
Snacks for the Lunchroom Fridge

Many workplaces have refrigerators and even kitchens in which to store your food. This list focuses on perishables that make for nutritious grazing.

Applesauce, unsweetened
Half sandwich
Leftovers
Low- or nonfat cottage cheese
Low- or nonfat yogurt
Nonfat cheese

One-minute meals (chapter 19)
Salad
Sliced chicken breast
Sliced turkey breast
Soup

CHOOSING THE RIGHT GRAZING FOODS

Many of my clients have a difficult time thinking about what to eat for snacks. To make it simple, I have compiled a list of snacks to fit your needs for any occasion.

A new listing of brand name snacks included in Table 2.1 will make it easier to get started without having to wade through thousands of food labels. (I will give quick tips for label reading in chapter 4.)

For more mini-meal ideas that take less than 60 seconds to fix, see chapter 19, ''Quickest: One-Minute Meals.''

Table 2.1 Brand Name Snacks Worth Grazing On

Food	Calories	Fat (g)	% Fat calories
Dairy			
Cheeses:			
Alpine Lace Free and Lean	35	trace	0
Knudsen flavored lowfat cottage cheese			
Peach	170	2	11

Food	Calories	Fat (g)	% Fat calories
Spiced apple/raisin	180	2	10
Strawberry	170	2	11
Kraft Free Singles (American)	45	0	0
Lifetime 1-oz nonfat snack cheese (cheddar, garden vegetable, mild Mexican, Swiss)	40	0	0

Fruit

Applesauce (no sugar), single-serve cups

Food	Calories	Fat (g)	% Fat calories
Mott's natural	50	0	0
Seneca	50	0	0
Weight Watchers Apple Chips	70	0	0
Weight Watchers fruit snacks (apple, cinnamon, strawberry, peach)	50	trace	0

Grains

Chips:

Food	Calories	Fat (g)	% Fat calories
Skinny Munchies (barbecue, onion, nacho)	59	2	30
Weight Watchers Corn Snackers	60	2	30
Weight Watchers Corn Snackers (nacho)	60	2	30

Crackers:

Food	Calories	Fat (g)	% Fat calories
Ak-mak	117	2	18
Carr's whole wheat	140	2	13
Nabisco Harvest Crisp	60	2	30
RyKrisp natural	40	0	0
RyKrisp seasoned	45	1	20
Wasa			
Fiber plus	35	1	26
Lite-rye	30	0	0
Sesame rye	30	1	30
Sesame wheat	60	2	30
Weight Watchers Crispbread	30	0	0
Grainfields snack-size cereal	70-120	0	0

Microwave Popcorn:

Food	Calories	Fat (g)	% Fat calories
Orville Redenbacher's Light	50	1	18
Weight Watchers	100	1	9
Popcorn rice cakes (all brands)	40	0	0
Rice cakes (all brands)	35	0	0

Meat/Alternatives

Food	Calories	Fat (g)	% Fat calories
Pop-top tuna (3-1/2 oz) (any brand packed in water)	126	2	14

Miscellaneous

Food	Calories	Fat (g)	% Fat calories
Jell-O-Light Pudding Snacks (chocolate or vanilla)	100	2	18

Light Balance Lunch Bucket:

Food	Calories	Fat (g)	% Fat calories
Beef Americana	190	3	14

(Cont.)

Table 2.1   (Continued)

Food	Calories	Fat (g)	% Fat calories
Beef and Pasta Bordeaux	180	1	5
Chicken Cacciatore	210	1	4
Chicken Fiesta	210	4	17
Pasta and Garden Vegetables	170	1	5
Mushroom Stroganoff	190	6	28
Vegetable juice (any brand)	40	0	0

CHAPTER

3

Eating on the Run Strategies

"I'm lucky to get home at night, let alone eat."—
accountant during tax season

Whether it is dashing through the door or off to another endless meeting, getting something to eat and keeping healthy is often the last thing on your mind. Rather it's another hassle, a chore. And like most chores, it's put off until the last moment.

Waiting until the last minute to decide about your eating may render you a victim of your environment, regardless of your honorable intentions. If you put your health at the bottom of your priority list, the consequences will inevitably catch up with you.

PLANNING

The secret to successful eating on the run is a little planning. Most people meticulously plan what they will do in a day, from whom they will see and what they will accomplish, to car tune-ups, golf games, manicures, and so forth. Yet, for some reason, when I mention planning (the "p" word) to patients, they grimace.

The barriers come up and the excuses fly as to why they don't plan their eating the same way they plan their daily schedule (even though they pride themselves on their organized appointment books).

Here are some typical excuses that may sound familiar to you:

"I have to wait until I'm hungry."

"I don't know where I will be."

"I don't have time to plan."

"I don't know how long my meetings will last."

"I'm in my car all day."

Don't worry. Your eating plan does not have to be rigid in structure. Actually, it should be quite the opposite: There must be flexibility built in. But you do need a foundation or framework from which to build.

Finding Time

Although chaos may seem to be your norm, or you feel like a slave to your appointment book, it's important to find time to eat something—be it snacks, mini-meals, or meals. Whether you're chasing deadlines or catching planes, most people have an idea of what the upcoming day will be like. Here's what you can do.

Identify Eating Opportunities. Ask yourself how you can best fit eating into your schedule. Some days, it may seem impossible. If that's the case, are there any times in which you could combine eating with another activity? For instance, you could eat while

- walking to your car, train, or plane;
- getting ready for work;
- driving or riding;
- working at your desk; or
- killing time between appointments.

Please note that ideally it would be good to sit down for 20 minutes and do nothing but eat and enjoy the food. But when you are in a time crunch, it's a matter of survival. It is better to fuel your body in a less-than-ideal setting than to go without eating.

Meal by Meal

The most difficult eating times seem to be breakfast and lunch. But dinner is the most challenging to plan because it seems too time-consuming.

Breakfast.   Don't leave home without it. The importance of a morning meal has already been sermonized. If you are not used to eating early, you may just need a little time to get adjusted. The best approach is to start simple. There's nothing wrong with leftovers. Or good old cereal and milk is easy and quick.

If for some reason even this seems too overwhelming, make sure you graze on a morning snack such as a lowfat muffin with nonfat milk. (For more ultraquick ideas, see chapter 19 with 40 mini-meals that take 60 seconds or less to make.)

Lunch.   Lunch hour? What's that? Many of my industrious clients work straight through lunch. "Looks good on the corporate résumé," they say. If they do decide to use their "hour," it is not usually for eating but for running errands.

If finding time for lunch presents a problem, try brown bagging or throw some wholesome snacks into your briefcase. Keep healthy grazing foods stocked in the corporate kitchen. (Eating out and fast food are addressed in upcoming chapters.)

According to the Brown Bag Institute, more than 55% of adults in the United States take their lunch to work. Brown bagging also has the advantage of "being there." The food is readily available for you to graze on all day long if you don't have time for a real lunch break.

When possible, I highly recommend eating away from your desk or workplace for the following reasons:

- It helps clear the mind.
- It gives you a rest that will enhance your productivity.
- It's a good stress breaker.
- It's more enjoyable and satisfying.
- It will make you a more conscious eater.

On days when you are rushed, you may want to try eating alone rather than with co-workers. If you take a book with you, that's usually a polite cue that you want to be alone and generally you will not be disturbed.

Dinner.   Just thinking about dinner meals sounds exhausting, especially after a long day.

A frequent scenario is to come home and gaze into the refrigerator or cupboards, as if waiting for something to magically appear. You finally decide (a feat in itself) that spaghetti sounds good, but you find your cupboards are bare—and your stomach is rumbling. By this time you settle for anything. Tonight it's popcorn for dinner. Sound familiar?

Such torture. Day after day, endlessly waiting for inspiration. Not only is this tiresome, it wastes your precious time. Here's one solution that works.

5 in 5 Approach

This is the technique that I have found the most effective and easiest to use (for my patients and myself). Since planning dinner was always such an obstacle, I routinely began to ''make'' people plan their meals in my office.

I would merely have my patients plan five dinner meals. Meanwhile I was secretly timing them! When they finished planning (only the main entrée, which is the core problem area), I would announce how long it took. On the average it would take 5 minutes or less to plan five meals. Easy! And to think they would often waste 10 minutes or more daily trying to come up with something to eat for dinner.

Why plan five meals rather than a whole week (seven meals)? It has been my experience that, between leftovers and eating out, five meals will easily stretch into a week's worth of eating.

By the way, please do not feel obligated to have chicken on Monday, chili on Tuesday, and so on (that would be rigid). Just select any meal from your list.

Of course, make sure you have the ingredients on hand. Ideally you would shop for groceries based on that list.

Catching 5 Minutes to Plan.   It's easy to grab 5 minutes to plan five meals. Do it while

- waiting for a meeting to start;
- waiting in line;
- waiting for an appointment; or
- waiting anywhere.

Once you have your meal list, post it somewhere convenient.

The Quickest 5 in 5.   To save more time, try making a master list of any and all meals you would be willing to prepare (and eat). Use the master list to plan the five meals. It won't require any thinking, just choosing.

Grazing

Plan for grazing on days that you are likely to go many hours between meals, or on days you work particularly long hours. Remember, skipping meals or going several hours without eating could result in unplanned rampages at vending machines, catering trucks, or doughnut platters (routinely available at meetings), or in gorging at dinner.

Minicase: I had a client who was having difficulty losing weight and often complained of fatigue. She said of her typical day, "I'm so busy getting the kids ready in the morning that I usually don't eat. Then I run errands. By the time I get home, it's too late to eat lunch, so I wait until dinner." You could by now guess her problem: gorging at dinner and fatigue from going too long without eating. The solution: two grazing snacks—midmorning and afternoon—planned within the framework of three small meals. She not only lost weight, but her lethargy disappeared.

NUTRITION ROAD MAP: QUALITY CONTROL

The only other step to planning, besides making time, is to consider what to eat. Your selections should be within the 6-5-4-3-2 Nutrition Countdown. Are you getting 6 grain servings, 5 fruit or vegetable servings, and so forth by the end of the day?

CONTROLLING YOUR ENVIRONMENT

All the planning efforts in the world do little good if they are not backed by action and supplies (food).

The easiest action is to take control of your eating environment. This means shopping for the right foods and having them on hand when you need them. Here are the essentials:

1. Routinely shop (rather than haphazardly running to the store, which costs you more time).
2. If you hate to grocery shop try
   - taking advantage of grocery stores that will assemble your food (all you have to do is call or fax in your order) or
   - using an errand service or a high school kid to shop for you.
3. You should have a planned grocery list; this will save oodles of time.
4. Don't forget to keep healthy staples in your cupboard so that you always have a good food choice on hand. This is especially important if you graze frequently.

While you are getting used to the idea of planning and routine grocery shopping, you may want to refer to the one-week Eating on the Run plan in chapter 20. This plan, which includes a shopping list, may serve as a nice buffer.

4

Avoiding Traps in the Grocery Store

"I put off grocery shopping until my cupboards are bare."—

marketing executive working 60-hour weeks

Do you dread grocery shopping? For most people it ranks right up there with doing the dishes or the laundry. I must confess that I, too, do not relish shopping for groceries. My husband and I take turns trying to outbribe each other into going. Ironically, I do enjoy spending time in the supermarket examining new foods and labeling trends.

In our haste to get grocery shopping over and done with, it's easy to unintentionally buy the wrong kinds of foods. Healthy-sounding labels can disguise high-fat, low-nutrition foods. For example,

"95% fat-free"—can be high in fat calories (whole milk is 96% fat-free by weight but contains nearly 50% fat calories);

"contains oat bran"—can mean anything since there is no legal definition of how much oat bran foods labeled as such must contain.

Some convenience foods have an undeserved healthy reputation, and when you're too busy to study the label, you might be fooled by this halo effect. Sure, popcorn is a great snack, but most microwave versions are rich in fat and salt. Likewise, turkey is a very lean meat, but processed into bologna it's just another fatty food. One turkey weiner can have 9 grams of fat and 80% fat calories.

And some foods just seem innocent. For example, Maruchan's Instant Lunch (soup with noodles) has up to 310 calories, 44% fat, and 1,750 milligrams of sodium. The National Academy of Sciences recommends a limit for sodium of 2,400 milligrams for the entire day! (See Table 4.1 for examples of the worst convenience foods.)

Table 4.1   Among the Worst Convenience Foods

Here is a selected listing of convenience foods that may surprise you with their high fat and sodium contents.

Food	Calories	Fat (g)	% Fat calories	Sodium (mg)
Beans:				
Armour				
Chili, No Beans	390	31	72	1,150
Chili with Beans	390	26	60	1,190
Hot Chili with Beans	390	25	58	1,190
Texas Chili with Beans	370	26	63	1,270
Dennison's				
Chili Con Carne with Beans	340	17	45	1,050
Cook-Off Chili with Beans	340	19	50	915
Diet Foods:				
Figurines Diet Bars	100	5-6	45-54	220-240
"Helper" Meals (as prepared):				
Hamburger (most varieties)	300-390	14-22	37-55	840-1,740
Tuna				
Potpie	420	27	58	890
Salad	420	27	58	870
Meats (canned):				
Armour				
Corned Beef Hash	390	27	62	1,430
Deviled Ham	110	9	74	380
Vienna Sausages	170-200	16-18	80-85	390-750
Swanson				
Chunky Chicken Spread	60	4	60	140
Mixin' Chunk-style Chicken	130	8	55	230

(Cont.)

Table 4.1 (Continued)

Foods	Calories	Fat (g)	% Fat calories	Sodium (mg)
Microwave Specialties:				
Dennison's Chili Con Carne without				
Beans	310	19	55	1,310
Hormel Micro Cup				
Beef Stew	190	9	43	860
Chili Mac	200	10	45	1,040
Lasagna	250	13	47	1,060
Noodles and Chicken	180	8	40	1,000
Scalloped Potatoes with Ham	260	16	55	810
Lunch Buckets				
Chili Mac	260	13	45	1,370
Chili with Beans	340	16	42	1,210
Scalloped Potatoes	250	12	43	830
Top Shelf				
Linguine	350	19	49	1,300
Salisbury Steak	340	19	50	850
Miscellaneous:				
Oscar Mayer Lunchables	340-460	18-33	48-65	1,350-1,980
Louis Rich Lunch Breaks	380-420	22-29	52-62	1,595-1,875
Salads:				
Salad Singles				
Crabmeat Flavored	150	7	42	860
Seafood	160	9	51	810
Tuna	150	9	54	610
Suddenly Salad				
Caesar	170	8	42	450
Creamy Macaroni	200	10	45	280
Pasta Primavera	190	10	47	340
Ranch and Bacon	210	11	47	320
Underwood				
Chicken Salad	170	11	58	590
Ham Salad	180	13	65	890
Soups:				
Hearty Cup O'Noodles	290-300	13-15	40-47	1,100-1,250
Cup O'Noodles	270-300	12-14	39-43	1,200-1,900
Top Ramen/Oodles of Noodles	390-400	18	41-42	1,810-1,920

Cardinal rule: Never assume.

To save you time and aggravation, I am going to give you quick guidelines to get past the advertising hype. Then, for easy shopping, I'll give you a list of food staples you may want to keep on hand.

QUICK SHOPPING SURVIVAL: LABELS

I know you are busy, but I cannot emphasize enough how important it is to read a food label. Don't get stung by the puffed-up tidbits of nutritional trivia printed in big type. Recent legislation will require nutritional labeling on most foods and set definitions for ambiguous terms such as *light*. But shoppers should still beware. Here are some tips on what to look for when you read a food label.

- *First.* Ignore the front of the food label! It's just window dressing. Instead turn to the nutritional information.
- *Fat.* If you do nothing else, always check the fat (think of it as always checking the oil under your hood). There should be no more than 3 grams of fat for every 100 calories:

  3 grams fat/100 calories.

  This quick little formula will keep you just under 30% fat calories, without getting bogged down with heavy fat math. (For you fat-math buffs, 1 gram of fat has 9 calories.)
- *Sodium.* A food is considered low in sodium if it has 140 milligrams or less of sodium per serving. Aim for no more than 2,400 milligrams of sodium each day.
- *Sugar.* Cereals will usually provide information on sugar content. Less than 5 grams (about 1 teaspoon of sugar) per serving is acceptable.
- *Fiber.* Foods that contain 3 grams or more of dietary fiber can be considered good fiber sources.

TEN WAYS TO SPEED UP SHOPPING

Most of us consider grocery shopping to be an unpleasant chore. We hate fighting the crowds, waiting in line at the checkout counter, unloading, and putting away our haul once we return home. We always seem to buy more than we originally intend. Most of all, the whole process seems terribly time-consuming! Here are 10 timesaving tips to get you in and out of the grocery store quickly:

1. Always use a list.
2. Arrange your list according to aisle locations.
3. Avoid trouble aisles such as the candy aisle.
4. Don't bother tasting samples. They're time wasters designed to trap you into buying something you don't want or need.
5. Bring only cash (saves time at the checkout and saves you from temptation).
6. Divide and conquer: Divvy up the grocery list with someone else (such as your spouse, roommate, or kids).
7. Stock up on staples to cut down on trips.
8. Shop at a familiar store.
9. Shop during nonpeak hours (many stores are open 24 hours).
10. Consolidate your buying to one store rather than several specialty shops.

QUICK PICKS: AISLE BY AISLE

There are nearly 26,000 items to choose from in a typical grocery store. How perplexing! Here are some pointers to guide you, arranged by food categories for speed.

Dairy Case.

- *Milk*: Select nonfat, 1%, or 2% milk.
- *Cheese:* Choose cheeses with less than 5 grams of fat per ounce. If no nutritional information is available, buy cheeses made from part-skim milk. Try nonfat or lowfat cottage cheese. Here are some good lowfat brands: Alpine Lace, Borden's Lite Line, Kraft Light, Laughing Cow (reduced), Lifetime, Mini Bonbel (reduced), and Weight Watchers.
- *Yogurt:* Choose nonfat or lowfat yogurts.
- *Margarine:* Go for the lowest fat versions, usually diet or light. Buy the tub version (there's less saturated fat in this form). The lowest fat margarine spread available commercially is Heart Beat, by Nucoa, with only 25 calories per tablespoon. (Weight Watchers has 50 calories per tablespoon.)

Deli Case.

- *Luncheon meats:* Choose meats that have 2 grams of fat or less per serving.
- *Hot dogs:* Pass them up. Even the turkey and chicken versions are loaded with fat.
- *Fresh pasta:* This is a quick cooking alternative. But limit filled pastas, such as tortellini or ravioli; they may be high in fat.

Meat Case.
Choose the leanest.

- *Beef:* The three leanest cuts are top round, eye of round, and round tip.
- *Chicken:* Buy skinless, or remove skin.
- *Fish:* Avoid breaded and prefried.
- *Pork:* Select tenderloin or Canadian bacon (rather than regular bacon).
- *Turkey:* Beware of processed cuts such as turkey bologna.

Breads and Cereals.

- *Bread:* A whole grain should be the first ingredient, and 2 grams of fat per slice is the maximum. Include bagels, pita bread, and English muffins.
- *Bread products:* Beware of high-fat breads: croissants, pastries, doughnuts, biscuits, and scones.
- *Cereals:* Choose cereals with at least 4 grams of fiber and less than 5 grams of sugar per serving.
- *Crackers:* Buy lowfat crackers. Beware of fatty crackers such as Ritz or Triscuits.

Canned Foods.

- *Beans:* Stock up on beans. Even canned pork and beans are low in fat (only 2 to 3 grams of fat per serving). Vegetarian refried beans are also low in fat.
- *Fruit:* Select only those labeled "packed in own juice," or "no sugar added." Beware of light syrup—it has added sugar.
- *Juice:* Tomato or vegetable juice is a quick way to meet your vegetable quota. (But these juices are also high in salt, so don't become overly reliant on "liquid vegetables.") Make sure fruit juice is 100% juice (rather than a sugar beverage with a hint of juice).
- *Soups:* Steer clear of cream soups. Instead, choose broth-based varieties such as minestrone, chicken noodle, and vegetarian

vegetable. Look for lower salt varieties if you're watching your sodium intake.

Produce. You can't go wrong here. Load up. Try the convenient packed, fresh vegetables (they're washed and ready-to-go).

Miscellaneous.

- *Peanut butter:* Buy a natural-style brand such as Laura Scudders, and pour off the oil.
- *Tuna:* Buy water-packed.
- *Frozen desserts:* Stick with 100% juice bars, sorbet, frozen yogurt, and light ice creams that have 5 grams of fat or less per serving (that's 1 scoop or 1/2 cup).

Frozen meals. Frozen foods are a category of their own. The next entire chapter is devoted to them.

Now that you've got a quick idea of what to look for when grocery shopping, be sure to keep your kitchen stocked. It's a key to successful eating on the run. Shop from List 4.1 and the snacking lists in chapter 2 for a good supply of healthy food staples.

List 4.1
Stocking Up: Grocery Staples

Beans
  All varieties, dried
  Canned, plain
Dairy
  Lowfat cheeses (less than 5 g fat/oz)
    Alpine Lace
    Borden Lite Line
    Kraft Light
    Laughing Cow Reduced
    Lifetime
    Mini Bonbel Reduced
    Weight Watchers
  Nonfat or lowfat cottage cheese
  Nonfat or lowfat milk
  Nonfat or lowfat ricotta cheese
  Nonfat yogurt
Fruits/Vegetables
  All fresh
  Any plain frozen
  Canned tomatoes

  Dried fruits
  100% fruit juice
  Tomato sauce
  Vegetable juice
Grains
  Brown rice
  Flour
  Hot cereal
  Kashi
  Pasta
  Whole grain breads
  Whole grain cereal
  Whole grain crackers
Meats/Alternatives
  Chicken
  Fish
  Ground turkey
  Tofu
  Tuna, water-packed

5

Your Frozen Assets

"My idea of cooking after a long day is to shove a frozen dinner in the microwave."—

client

Zap. Dinner's on. Do you find yourself turning to frozen meals as a cure for kitchen fatigue syndrome? Or do you use them for the convenience of not having to wash dishes?

AVOIDING THE TRAPS

With the proliferation of microwaves (nearly eight in ten homes and half of all businesses have one), frozen entrées seem like an easy answer. But they can be a mixed blessing and even a nutritional nightmare, if you are not careful. The good news is that frozen meals can be part of a nutritious diet if you know what to look for and what to steer clear of. First, let's look at some common pitfalls you'll want to avoid: fat traps, salt mines, and other nutritional dilemmas.

Light Meals

The fastest growth in the frozen dinner business has been in the low-calorie segment, with sales in the billion dollar range. Foods labeled "light" or "lean" are not necessarily nutritious, nor are they necessarily low in fat.

Never assume a "slim" frozen meal is low in fat. A meal that supplies 300 calories (which seems to be the industry gold standard for a low-calorie entrée) can still be high in fat. For example, Lean Cuisine salisbury steak draws 48% of its calories from fat, and Weight Watchers cheese enchiladas ranchero has 45% fat calories. (See Table 5.1 for more examples.) Recall the healthy range we're aiming for is 30% fat calories.

Clearly, if you want your calories to count, you do not want to load them with fat. Especially since studies show that the amount of fat may be more important than total calories when trying to lose weight and keep it off. Fortunately, some frozen entrées are healthy. Table 5.2 has a long list of best bets by brand names. To compare how your favorite light frozen entrée measures up, refer to Appendix A for more details.

Table 5.1 "Light" but Heavy in Fat

Entrée	Calories	Fat (g)	% Fat calories	Sodium (mg)	Cholesterol (mg)
Budget Gourmet Light:					
Chicken Au Gratin	250	11	40	870	50
Chicken Enchiladas Suiza	290	12	37	810	40
Sirloin Salisbury Steak	260	13	45	700	65
Dining Lite:					
Fetuccini with Broccoli	290	12	37	1,020	35
Lean Cuisine:					
Salisbury Steak	280	15	48	840	100
Stuffed Cabbage	220	10	41	930	55
Mrs. Paul's:					
Crunchy Light Batter					
Fish Fillets	310	17	49	810	n/a
Fish Sticks	240	13	49	590	n/a
Flounder	310	16	47	790	n/a
Haddock	330	17	46	670	n/a
Supreme Light Batter Fish	210	12	51	540	n/a
Weight Watchers:					
Beef Enchiladas Ranchero	230	10	39	720	40
Cheese Enchiladas Ranchero	360	18	45	900	60
Chicken Cordon Bleu	220	9	37	630	50
Chicken Nuggets	270	12	40	540	50
Southern Fried Chicken Patty	320	16	45	690	65

n/a = data not available.

Table 5.2   Best Bets by Brand (Frozen Entrées)

This list offers only a few best bets for each brand. Refer to Appendix A for more.

Entrée	Cal-ories	Fat (g)	% Fat calories	Sodium (mg)	Cholesterol (mg)
Armour Classics:					
Chicken and Noodles	230	7	27	660	50
Chicken Fettucini	260	9	31	660	50
Armour Classics Lite:					
Beef Stroganoff	250	6	22	510	55
Chicken àla King	290	7	22	630	55
Chicken Burgundy	210	2	9	780	45
Chicken Oriental	180	1	5	660	35
Steak Diane	290	9	28	440	80
Banquet Dinners:					
Spaghetti and Meatballs	290	10	31	580	30
Budget Gourmet:					
Chicken Marsala	270	8	26	700	95
Pepper Steak with Rice	330	10	27	600	30
Sweet and Sour Chicken	340	5	13	630	40
Budget Gourmet Light Dinners:					
Teriyaki Chicken	290	9	28	780	35
Budget Gourmet Light Entrées:					
Cheese Lasagna with Vegetables	290	9	28	780	15
Glazed Turkey	270	5	17	760	40
Mandarin Chicken	300	7	21	670	40
Orange Glazed Chicken	250	3	11	350	10
Budget Gourmet 3-Dish:					
Scallops and Shrimp Marinara	330	9	25	730	70
Dining Lite:					
Cheese Lasagna	260	6	21	800	30
Chicken àla King	240	7	26	780	40
Chicken Chow Mein	180	2	10	650	30
Chicken with Noodles	240	7	26	570	50
Glazed Chicken	220	4	16	680	45
Lasagna with Meat Sauce	240	5	19	800	25
Healthy Choice Dinners:					
Chicken Oriental	220	2	8	460	55
Mesquite Chicken	310	2	6	270	45
Shrimp Creole	210	1	4	560	65

(Cont.)

Table 5.2 (Continued)

Entrée	Cal- ories	Fat (g)	% Fat calories	Sodium (mg)	Cholesterol (mg)
Shrimp Marinara	220	1	4	320	50
Sweet and Sour Chicken	280	2	6	260	50
Healthy Choice Entrées:	200-310	2-7	7-17	90-440	15-55
Kraft Eating Right:					
Chicken Breast and Vegetables	200	4	18	570	30
Glazed Chicken Breast	240	4	15	560	35
Lasagna with Meat Sauce	270	7	23	440	30
Shrimp Vegetable Stir Fry	150	4	24	400	50
Swedish Meatballs	290	7	22	470	55
Lean Cuisine:					
Breast of Chicken Marsala	190	5	24	400	80
Cheese Pizza (French Bread)	310	10	29	750	15
Chicken a l'Orange	260	5	17	430	55
Filet of Fish Divan	260	7	24	750	85
Sliced Turkey Breast in Mushroom Sauce	240	7	26	790	50
Lean Pockets:					
Beef and Broccoli	250	8	29	760	n/a
Chicken Parmesan	270	6	20	750	n/a
Pizza Deluxe	280	9	29	500	n/a
Legume:					
Manicotti Florentine	260	7	24	650	0
Mexican Enchiladas	270	8	27	390	0
Vegetable Lasagne	240	8	30	520	0
Le Menu Healthy Dinners:					
Cheese Tortellini	230	6	23	460	15
Glazed Chicken	230	3	12	480	55
Sliced Turkey	210	5	21	540	30
Turkey Divan	260	7	24	420	60
Veal Marsala	230	3	12	700	75
Mrs. Paul's Light Seafood:					
Fish Dijon	200	5	23	650	60
Seafood Lasagna	290	8	25	750	57
Seafood Rotini	240	6	23	570	25
Shrimp and Clams with Linguini	240	5	19	750	40
Shrimp Cajun Style	230	5	20	740	60
Swanson:					
Sweet and Sour Chicken	380	11	26	520	n/a

Entrée	Cal-ories	Fat (g)	% Fat calories	Sodium (mg)	Cholesterol (mg)
Tyson (chicken):					
A l'Orange	300	8	24	670	n/a
Mesquite	320	10	28	700	n/a
Ultra Slim Fast:					
Beef Pepper Steak and Parsleyed Rice	270	4	14	690	45
Mesquite Chicken	360	1	3	300	65
Pasta Primavera	340	9	24	730	25
Shrimp Creole	240	4	15	730	80
Sweet and Sour Chicken	330	2	6	340	45
Weight Watchers:					
Cheese Tortellini	310	6	17	570	15
Chicken Divan Baked Potato	280	4	13	730	40
Ham Lorraine Baked Potato	250	4	14	670	15
Imperial Chicken	240	3	11	640	35
Sweet 'n Sour Chicken Tenders	240	1	4	600	40

n/a = data not available.

Healthy-Sounding but Not

Chicken- and fish-based meals are always a healthy choice, right? Wrong. Some traditional standbys, such as chicken potpie or fish sticks, can be oozing with fat (which cancels out the naturally low-in-fat characteristics of fish and chicken). For example, a chicken potpie may have 410 to 630 calories, depending on the brand. To make matters worse, most of these calories come from fat. One brand of chicken potpie has the equivalent of 9 teaspoons of fat in 1 serving. To see how your favorite standbys rate, check Table 5.3 for data on healthy-sounding but fatty frozen meals.

Salt Mines

Light in calories does not necessarily mean light in sodium either. Most frozen meals have a high sodium content. Depending on the

Table 5.3 Healthy-Sounding but Fatty Frozen Meals

Entrée	Calories	Fat (g)	% Fat calories	Sodium (mg)	Cholesterol (mg)
Armour Classics:					
Chicken Parmigiana	370	19	46	1,060	75
Glazed Chicken	300	16	48	960	60
Banquet Dinners:					
Chicken and Dumplings	430	24	50	940	45
Turkey Dinner	390	20	46	1,110	40
Banquet Extra Helpings:					
Chicken Nuggets Dinner with					
Barbecue Sauce	640	36	51	1,390	n/a
Budget Gourmet:					
Chicken and Egg Noodles	440	25	51	980	100
Shrimp with Fettuccine	370	22	54	750	140
Hungry Man Dinners:					
Boneless Chicken	700	28	36	1,530	n/a
Fried Chicken (White Meat)	870	46	48	2,150	n/a
Hungry Man Potpies:					
Chicken	630	35	50	1,600	n/a
Turkey	650	36	50	1,470	n/a
Le Menu:					
Chicken Kiev	530	39	66	780	n/a
Chicken Parmigiana	410	20	44	1,030	n/a
Swanson:					
Chicken Nibbles	340	20	53	730	n/a
Chicken Pie	410	21	46	1,030	n/a
Stouffer's:					
Barbecue-Style Chicken	390	23	53	1,250	n/a
Chicken Pie	530	33	56	1,260	n/a
Lobster Newburg	380	32	76	870	n/a
Pasta Carbonara	620	45	65	780	n/a
Pasta Primavera	270	21	70	580	n/a
Tortellini with Vinaigrette dressing	400	27	61	540	n/a
Turkey Pie	540	36	60	1,300	n/a
Tyson:					
Chicken Français	280	14	45	1,130	n/a
Chicken Kiev	520	33	57	1,200	n/a
Peking Chicken	390	20	46	860	n/a

n/a = data not available.

brand and type of entrée, you could end up with a shakerful of sodium. Even the health-conscious entrées are not low-sodium, although they are within acceptable ranges. Here are some glaring examples of salt mines:

- Stouffer's entrées have up to 1,920 milligrams sodium.
- Hungry Man Dinners have up to 2,150 milligrams sodium.
- Great Starts Breakfast on a Biscuit has up to 1,850 milligrams sodium.

Other Traps and Myths

1. Beware of terms such as "lightly breaded." This usually translates into lightly fried, and you will still get a substantial dose of fat. Most breaded entrées have been deep-fried, but you can't see or feel the greasy texture when it is frozen.
2. Hungry Man meals (and other similar brands) should really be called "Fatty Man" or "Sodium Man." Not only do you get larger or extra portions, you also get a heap of extra unwanted fat and sodium.
3. Most frozen dinners are not complete meals. They still require a little planning to assure a balanced day of eating. This is especially true for entrée-only meals that come with no added vegetables or accompaniments.
4. Frozen meals are typically lacking in calcium, vitamins A and C, and fiber. (But you can easily fortify these deficits through a grazing approach.)

CHOOSING CAREFULLY

Cheer up. A new trend in healthy frozen entrées is developing in which food manufacturers are attempting to meet health goals consistently (rather than solving one nutritional problem while creating another). Examples of these brands include Healthy Choice by Con Agra and Kraft Eating Right. These entrées are lower in fat, calories, cholesterol, and sodium.

Still, it's a good idea to read the label, so you can be sure of what you're getting. Ideally there should be no more than

- 3 grams of fat for every 100 calories (roughly 30% fat calories);
- 800 milligrams of sodium (this is one third of the National Academy of Sciences' recommended maximum sodium intake of 2,400 milligrams a day); and

- 100 milligrams of cholesterol (again, one third of the National Academy of Sciences' recommended maximum intake of cholesterol).

Also, keep the following general tips in mind:

- Oriental-style meals tend to be lower in fat and calories.
- Cheese-sauce dishes are usually high in fat and calories.
- Potpies are usually high in fat and calories.
- Plain frozen vegetables are an easy nutritional bargain.
- Salisbury steaks generally have excessive fat.
- Any breaded pieces or parts of chicken or fish are usually trouble.
- Hearty-man types of meals are best avoided.
- Other frozen entrées, such as breakfast meals, tend to be high in fat, sodium, and cholesterol. (There are exceptions. See Table 5.4 for best bets in frozen breakfast foods.)

Table 5.4   Best Bets in Frozen Breakfasts

Entrée	Calories	Fat (g)	% Fat calories	Sodium (mg)	Cholesterol (mg)
Pillsbury:					
Microwave Pancakes	240-260	4	14-15	420-590	n/a
Weight Watchers:					
Canadian Bacon and Cheese Muffin	240	8	30	610	n/a
Pancakes	230-250	4	14-16	430	n/a
Swanson Great Starts:					
Egg and Cheese on Bagel	240	8	30	670	n/a
Ham and Cheese on Bagel	220	6	25	630	n/a
Jimmy Dean Microwave:					
Ham and Cheese Muffin	130	4	28	480	n/a

n/a = data not available.

Note. From "Frozen Breakfast Entrees: Convenience at a Cost" by B. Weinstein, 1990, *Environmental Nutrition,* **13**(4), p. 4. Copyright 1990 by Larry Goldblatt. Reprinted with permission from the Environmental Nutrition Newsletter, 2112 Broadway, Suite 200, New York, NY 10023.

MAXIMIZING YOUR FROZEN ASSETS

To round out your frozen meal with a nutrition boost, add one or more of the following:

- Nonfat, 1% fat, or 2% fat milk
- Whole grain bread or whole grain crackers
- Raw vegetables
- Plain (no sauce), microwavable frozen vegetables
- Fresh fruit
- Corn tortilla
- Simple salad

You may also want to consider making your own easy-to-do frozen meals. (See chapters 18, 19, and 20 for lots of ideas.)

6

Best Bets in Restaurant Row

"I eat out every day, at least two out of three meals."—
sales representative

We have entered the Era of Dash Dining, according to one columnist for the trade magazine *Restaurant Hospitality*. Once considered a luxury, eating out has evolved into a daily lifestyle, considered essential by many.

Be it an occupational requirement or pure enjoyment, no other area of eating seems as challenging as eating out. If you are not careful, eating out could easily wreak havoc on your waistline and arteries. Consider that one out of five meals are eaten away from home, but over one third of total calories are consumed when eating out.

The first step to healthy (but still tasty) dining is to "have it your way." Yet, many people feel awkward making special requests. However, it is only because of special requests that lowfat milk, for example, is now routinely available in restaurants.

I have also had patients feel that it would be too much of a "scene" to make requests. But it does not have to be a big production. Just matter-of-factly make your requests, or ask how a food is prepared. There is no need to announce that your cholesterol or weight is high or go into a long spiel.

YOUR RESTAURANT RIGHTS

Remember that the restaurant business is a service industry. They want to meet your needs, or they could go out of business. Also, many special requests are very simple for the restaurant to do. Get into the habit of having food served your way. Here are a few special requests to get you started:

- Lowfat milk instead of cream for coffee
- Sauces and dressings on the side
- Whole grain bread
- Extra plate (to split an entrée)
- Remove the skin from the chicken
- Broiled dry
- Fresh fruit or small green salad instead of french fries
- Hold the butter
- Lemon wedges or gourmet vinegar for salad dressing
- Baked potato instead of french fries
- Steamed vegetables plain rather than with butter

Remember, you are the valued customer. You pay the bill and have the right to

- ask how food is prepared;
- request that a food be fixed differently (broiled or hold the sauce);
- send food back if it has not been prepared satisfactorily;
- ask for items not listed on the menu (such as lemon for your salad);
- request a doggie bag, even before the food is served;
- bring your own special condiments such as diet dressing;
- call the restaurant ahead of time to request that your food be prepared a special way;
- ask any question without fear of embarrassment or the "evil eye" from the waiter or waitress;
- leave if the restaurant cannot or does not wish to accommodate your needs; and
- expect special service—every customer is important.

RESTAURANT HEALTH AID KIT

Even restaurants willing to meet your requests may not be able to accommodate 100% of your needs, so be prepared with a restaurant health aid kit. Simply keep a portable supply of "essentials" such as

- Butter Buds or Molly McButter,
- diet dressings,
- herbal tea bags,
- sodium-free seasoning/herbs,
- sugar substitute (most restaurants do carry this), and
- Weight Watchers Dairy Creamer (packets of instant nonfat dry milk).

FOUR KEY STRATEGIES

There are many ways to stay ahead of the eating-out game without feeling deprived. First, keep in mind these core guidelines to assure your success wherever you dine and no matter how frequently you eat out.

Leave Food on the Plate.   Combine the generous servings of most restaurants with the clean-plate consciousness of most people, and you have double trouble—more calories and more fat than you need at one meal. Consider, for example, that most restaurants serve two chicken breasts (double the meat you need) and a petite steak is usually 8 ounces. These entrées easily exceed the recommended maximum of seven ounces of animal protein daily. If you eat out often, this can obviously be a problem.

Breaking the clean-plate habit, especially when eating out, is probably one of the most important steps you can take. Even if you are dining out at the fattiest French restaurant in town (Chez à la Grease), leaving half the food behind rids you of half the fat calories.

By now most of you know the fallacies of belonging to the clean-plate club. Yet, as often as you begin a restaurant meal with good intentions, you still wind up eating everything. Try the following helpful tricks that have helped many of my clients (and me).

- Put your napkin on the plate when you're done; don't wait until your plate is empty. This will signal the waiter that you have finished your meal, and usually the plate will be removed promptly. Also, a napkin on your plate prevents unintentional nibbling as your conversation meanders (you are not going to dig under the napkin for food).
- Place your fork and knife entirely over your plate and be sure the handles are touching the remaining food. This too will prevent innocent nibbling—no one wants to pick up a wet, soiled utensil.
- Request a doggie bag before the meal is served. Simply put half of your food in the bag when your meal arrives. Out of sight, out of mind.

Control Where You Eat. Whether you are eating alone or with a group of people, it usually takes a little time and planning to decide where to eat. And where you eat can determine what you eat. You can influence a group decision with the power of suggestion. Be prepared to name a couple of restaurants that have at least one healthy entrée that you enjoy.

Don't Get Caught in the Get-Your-Money's-Worth Trap. Regardless of economic background there is something tempting about getting more than your money's worth when it comes to food. Ever find yourself eating a lot of food to make sure you get a good deal? At the increasingly popular buffets, salad bars, and brunches, it is very easy to eat more than enough.

Put the value on your health rather than on the quantity of food you consume. It is no bargain if years of gluttonous eating of fatty foods results in bypass surgery. Exaggeration? Maybe. But why take the chance?

Never Assume. I am still surprised at the mistakes that I, a nutritionist, can make. Let me describe a few to you to save you from the same folly.

I arrived in Boston very late and ordered what I thought would be a light meal—broiled scallops. To my surprise, the scallops were broiled in butter! Usually a broiled item is cooked dry. A few days later in New York, I ordered a shrimp salad with dressing on the side. In California this would be either jumbo or bay shrimp on a bed of lettuce, but what I received was the equivalent of tuna salad—chopped shrimp heavy on the mayo. Yuck! Remember our cardinal rule: Never assume. Always ask how foods are prepared, even the basic items.

A HEALTHY ORDER

Believe it or not, you are not doomed to dull eating, nor do you have to be a party pooper when you order a healthy meal. In some restaurants, it's only a matter of selecting an entrée that already exists on the menu. For example, how do these tantalizing entrées sound? Deadly or healthy?

- Baked red snapper in shallot crust with orange leek sauce
- Tenderloin with red pepper and cilantro sauce
- Chicken brochetti

These mouth-watering dishes are examples of healthy entrées prepared by creative chefs from trendy restaurants. They are all under 300 calories and have 30% fat calories or less.

Just a few changes in your ordering style can make a big calorie difference without sacrificing fun and taste. Here's an example of how small changes made a big difference for Don, one of my clients.

Don had the pleasurable task of wining and dining potential new clients. However, this obligation brought with it the occupational hazard of weight gain.

His meals usually began with two rounds of drinks and ended with dessert. Don wanted to lose weight while maintaining his professional duties. We worked together using a problem-solving approach, introducing only realistic changes that he was *willing* to make. The end result was a bit staggering—a savings of approximately 1,612 calories in one meal. See Table 6.1 for the before-and-after analysis. As you can see, Don did not want to give up the sour cream for his potato, which turned out to be okay in the long run because he saved so many calories elsewhere. Don still has his steak and cheesecake occasionally, but he no longer puts stress on his body with a daily heavy dose of calories and fat. His weight dropped significantly, simply by making these few changes and without going on a "diet."

When you order a meal with your health at heart, it's disappointing to find out that your dinner is a diet disaster. Understanding restaurant menu jargon can help prevent that disheartening experience. Table 6.2 lists examples of menu jargon, including examples of key words for both lowfat and high-fat dishes. Typical healthy-sounding menu items that turn out to be fat traps are given in Table 6.3.

Table 6.1 Typical Restaurant Meal

Before	Calories	After	Calories
2 vodka collins	360	1 wine spritzer	80
		1 Perrier with twist	0
Fried mushrooms	156	Cucumber vinaigrette	10
10 oz steak, teriyaki	1,359	Chicken breast, teriyaki (skinless)	370
Large baked potato	139	Large baked potato	139
2 tbsp sour cream	52	2 tbsp sour cream	52
Buttered peas	115	Fresh steamed vegetables	25
Cheesecake	257	Angel food cake with fresh strawberries	150
TOTAL	**2,438**	**TOTAL**	**826**

Table 6.2   Menu Jargon

The food on a menu is usually described sumptuously to make your mouth water. Here are some key adjectives that could either help or hurt you.

Good choice (lowfat)	Least healthy choice (high-fat)
Steamed	Fried
Broiled	Crispy
Poached	Buttery, butter sauce
Garden fresh	Creamed
In its own juice	In its own gravy
Tomato sauce	Cream sauce
Roasted	Au gratin, cheese sauce
Marinated in juice or wine	Marinated in oil or butter
Charbroiled	Scampi style
Boiled	Breaded
Marinara	Meat sauce
Barbecued	Sautéed
Stir-fried	Alfredo
Mesquite-grilled	Pan-fried
Stuffed with vegetables	Stuffed with cheese

Table 6.3   Healthy-Sounding Fat Traps

Food	Problem
Breaded zucchini	Breaded usually means fried, which wipes out the lowfat veggie benefits.
Cobb salad	Fat traps galore: avocado, bacon, bleu cheese, olives, salad dressing.
Diet plate	Usually consists of cottage cheese, sirloin patty, and canned fruit. A fatty meal.
Quiche	Crust is loaded with fat. Cheese is a rich fat source. Many quiches also use cream.
Salad bar	Surprised? If you stick with the raw produce (fruits and vegetables), no problem. But creamy salads such as macaroni, potato, and pasta salad are oozing with fat. Accoutrements such as cheese, sunflower seeds, olives, avocados, bacon, and salad dressing can easily add up to a 1,000-calorie meal.
Seafood platter	Fish components are often fried. (Ask how it's prepared.)

COURSE BY COURSE

Despite the trend toward healthy menu options in restaurants, navigating your way through a menu can still be tricky. This section will highlight best bets and limitations of menu fare, course by course.

Appetizers

Consider making a main course out of your appetizer (the portion size would be just about right). Try ordering a dinner salad as the appetizer, followed by another appetizer such as pasta marinara.

Best Bets.   Fresh steamed vegetables, tomato juice, dinner salads, steamed or broiled seafood, seafood cocktails.

Best Limited.   Potato skins, pâté, fried vegetables, fried cheese, tortilla chips.

A special note about tortilla chips: The biggest problem here is the "can't have just one" syndrome. No matter how many times you push that chip basket away, your arm seems to find it. That magnetic phenomenon combined with the never empty basket (thanks to a good waiter or waitress) usually results in your being full by the time the meal arrives.

Chip solution: One approach is what I call the "allocation method." You allocate six chips to your bread plate. (I chose six because that roughly equals one tortilla.) Have all the salsa you want, but savor those chips because when they are gone—hasta la vista. The difference here is now you are conditioned to an empty bread plate as your stopping point, rather than the never-never land of the bottomless chip basket.

The other trick is the abstinence approach, which works well when you are among good friends or loved ones who also share the love-hate relationship with chips. You simply request that no chips be placed on your table.

Bread

If you arrive at a restaurant overly ravenous, it is best to request that the bread be served with the meal. If not, you may end up devouring all the rolls or fresh bread slices you can get your hands on.

Because bread is usually served hot (nice and moist), this is a good opportunity to cut down on butter or margarine. If you can't do without a spread, use jam or honey. They're lower in calories and have no fat.

Best Bets.   Whole grain bread, corn tortillas, flat breads.

Best Limited.   Croissants, muffins, biscuits, flour tortillas.

Salad

If you are not careful, your salad could easily drown in a fat bath. A few dollops from an industrial-size dressing ladle could pack a big calorie wallop. Those innocent-looking ladles carry about 2 ounces. Three plops could add up to 900 calories! (The average dressing has about 75 calories per tablespoon, and there are 2 tablespoons in an ounce.)

Best Bets.

1. Request dressing on the side and try the "fork-dip-stab" method. Dip your fork into the dressing and then stab your lettuce. You get flavor in every bite but far fewer calories. This may sound awkward, but it's really inconspicuous.
2. Request a soufflé cup (a small paper cup) when at a salad bar so that you can put your dressing on the side.
3. Try a zippy lemon wedge for a fat-free dressing.
4. Request a gourmet vinegar.
5. Choose a reduced-calorie dressing.

Best Limited.   Regular dressings; fatty salad add-ons such as olives, bacon, avocado, grated cheese. Request that these be left off.

Entrée

Generally, the KIS (Keep It Simple) approach works well here. Remember, never assume—ask how the entrée is prepared. Don't forget to inquire about the silent accompaniments that go with the entrée, such as the vegetables and side entrées. Do make special requests that are suitable for you.

Best Bets.

1. Request an extra plate and split an entrée with your dining partners.
2. See List 6.1 at the end of the chapter for specific best bets for international cuisines.
3. Don't forget to order your doggie bag in advance of the meal.

Best Limited. Cheese-based entrées, fried foods, large meat portions, potpies, quiches. All are loaded with fat.

Beverages

It is very easy to guzzle calories in innocent-sounding beverages, especially high-calorie alcoholic drinks.

If you anticipate drinking alcohol, set a limit in advance. Order wine by the glass rather than the liter, or you'll find it easy to drink more than you planned.

Best Bets. Juice, nonfat or lowfat milk, mineral water, spritzer. Request milk for your coffee instead of cream.

Best Limited. Regular sodas, milk shakes.

Dessert Tray

Unless you are a glutton for punishment, request that the dessert tray not be shown to you. That way you won't be tempted by those luscious desserts staring right at your mouth.

Best Bets. Try a gourmet dessert coffee or cappucino, and request that nonfat milk be used for steaming. In the mood to splurge? Order a dessert for the table with a round of forks. Usually one or two bites is very satisfying, especially after a meal. Other good dessert choices include sorbets, ices, angel food cake, fresh berries (sans cream), and nonfat frozen yogurt.

Best Limited. Most!

Breakfast

I consider ordering breakfast to be a special challenge. There seem to be fewer choices, and the choices available aren't that appealing. (I've often had clients balk at paying for a box of cold cereal and milk.)

Generally, you are better off to order à la carte because most dishes come with bacon, sausage, or hash browns (grease, grease, or grease).

I once ate breakfast with a reporter who was very curious to see what I would order. I chose three pancakes (no butter) and orange juice. The reporter was surprised that I did not hold the syrup. Nor do I recommend that practice to my clients. Why? The food needs to taste good! I know very few people who enjoy eating dry pancakes. Of course, I am not suggesting that you drown your hotcakes in syrup. When available, fresh strawberries or boysenberries are a healthy breakfast topping.

Best Bets.   Pancakes, French toast (request they be made with egg whites only—many restaurants can easily handle this request), fresh fruit platter, cold cereal, hot cereal, omelettes made with egg substitute, lox and bagels (with a minimum of cream cheese), whole wheat toast, plain bagels, fruit juice, tomato juice, vegetable juice. Remember to limit egg yolks to four per week and to hold the butter. Jam is a better choice than butter for a bread spread.

Best Limited.   The 2-2-2-2 type of meals (two eggs, two sausages, two pancakes, two strips of bacon). If you must have breakfast meat, Canadian bacon is an improvement. Also limit omelettes (unless made with egg substitutes or egg whites), croissants, biscuits, breakfast sandwiches.

Buffets and Salad Bars

Remember, your personal challenge is not to get more than your money's worth but to enjoy a health-smart meal.

Begin with a healthy mind-set. Consider brunches and buffets as simply a visual menu. For example, you don't order everything on the menu even if every item looks good, right? Similarly, you are not obligated to try everything on the buffet.

Best Bets.   Use a two-tiered approach to eating. This strategy requires making two trips (an appealing thought). On the first trip, help yourself to the raw fruits and vegetables. This high-fiber head start will provide bulk to take the edge off your hunger. And you'll be in better control of your food choices when you come back.

To cope with the food piling phenomenon, use the smallest plate available on the second trip. Get in the habit of taking taster-size portions. Remember the serving utensils are industrial size and it's easy to inadvertently wind up with a plate piled as high as Mount Everest.

Best Limited.

1. Overflowing champagne. After one round have the waiter or waitress remove your glass, or you may drink more than you want or need.

2. Goopy salads and casseroles. More often than not the goop that holds these foods together is fat, so go easy on these items or avoid them altogether.
3. Desserts. Desserts. Desserts. These tantalizing goodies are usually the first item you will face at a brunch, and they will often stay on your mind until you can hold out no longer. If dining with a group of people, have one dessert plate of samplers. You share the calories and reduce the guilt.
4. If you don't like it, don't eat it. Remember, rid yourself of the clean-plate mentality. In buffet situations, you will probably not be able to take advantage of a doggie bag. (Obviously, some people would abuse the courtesy and pre-bag a couple of meals.) The reality is that some food will go to waste. But better wasted, then w-a-i-s-t-e-d.

HEART-SMART RESTAURANTS

The American Heart Association (AHA) used to have a national restaurant program to assist diners in ordering heart-healthy meals. A tiny red heart next to an entrée on the menu meant the food conformed to AHA standards. Unfortunately, the AHA has discontinued the national program, but there is good news. A recent National Restaurant Association poll showed that nearly 40% of the restaurants surveyed offer menu items that are lower in calories, fat, and cholesterol. So it's getting easier to find heart-healthy items on the menu.

Bob's Big Boy, for example, has a "Health Smart" menu for all meals. To their credit, nutritional information is provided on the back of the menus, so there is no question as to what you are getting. Table 6.4 shows some promising examples from Bob's Big Boy of

Table 6.4   Healthy Foods From Bob's Big Boy

Menu item	Calories	Fat (g)	% Fat calories	Cholesterol (mg)
Cajun Cod*	438	14	29	89
Frozen Yogurt Shake	184	trace	0	0
Mushroom Omelette	332	6	16	0
Spaghetti Marinara*	450	6	15	8
Turkey Pita	224	5	20	75

*Includes a dinner salad (without dressing) and one slice of oat bran bread with margarine.

how healthy menu choices can be enticing without breaking your fat budget.

Lettuce Entertain You Enterprises, Inc. (LEYE), one of the nation's leading independent restaurant groups, is another shining example. For each of their 21 trendy restaurants, they created menu items that have 30% or less of their total calories from fat, yet these items "remain true to their restaurant's cuisine without sacrificing taste." LEYE goes one healthy step further; they provide healthy options for other courses—from appetizers to desserts. Whether you dine at Eccentric, Ed Debevic's, or any of LEYE's other popular restaurants, you will have a healthy choice, without sacrificing the fun of dining out or the enjoyment of food.

Take advantage of this healthy menu trend in restaurant dining. Remember, to stay in business, restaurants will do everything they can to meet your needs. You get to vote—with your fork and wallet!

GLOBAL EATING: ETHNIC FOOD

When ordering international cuisine, use the same food selection principles described earlier, but especially take care to ask what is in the food and how it is prepared. List 6.1 offers some specific best bets, adapted from Densie Webb's *International Cuisines Calorie Counter* and Hope Warshaw's *The Restaurant Companion*.

List 6.1
Best Bets in Ethnic Food

Chinese:

Appetizers/Accompaniments: chicken or vegetable lo mein, chicken won ton soup, hot and sour soup, sizzling rice soup (chicken or shrimp), spicy green beans, steamed Peking ravioli, steamed rice, subgum soup, vegetarian delight, velvet corn soup with crabmeat, won ton soup, Yu Hsiang eggplant

Entrées: chicken chop suey, delights of three, drunken chicken, mandarin pancakes, moo shu shrimp, Peking smoked chicken, shrimp with broccoli, shrimp with tomato sauce, sizzling sliced chicken, Szechuan seafood, teriyaki beef or chicken, velvet chicken lo mein, Yu Hsiang chicken

Dessert: lychee nuts

(Cont.)

List 6.1
(Continued)

Cajun:

Appetizers/Accompaniments: Cajun rice, candied yams, cornbread (no butter), fish sauce piquant, smothered potatoes, spicy tomatoes

Entrées: baked fresh fish with crabmeat gravy, beans with sausage and Cajun rice, crawfish boudin, shrimp and crabmeat jambalaya, shrimp and crabmeat spaghetti

Dessert: lemon coffee cake

French:

Appetizers/Accompaniments: baguette, egg bread, mold of parsleyed ham in aspic, purée of rice and turnips, spinach braised with onions, vegetables mélange

Entrées: huîtres fraîches, scallop bouillabaisse, steamed mussels, veal stew

Desserts: apples baked with rum, apricot sherbet, fresh raspberries with Chambord liqueur, fruits frais et sorbet, plums baked in custard, spice cake

Greek:

Appetizers/Accompaniments: baked beans plaki style, bean soup, chicken rice soup avgolemono, chick-pea soup, green beans braised with mint and potatoes, lentil soup, pita bread, tomatoes and herbs with rice, tzatsiki (cucumbers)

Entrées: lamb with artichokes and dill, plaki fish, shish kebab

Desserts: caramel custard, honey-cheese pie

Italian:

Appetizers/Accompaniments: chick-peas and pasta soup, marinated calimari, minestrone soup, steamed clams

Entrées: chicken cacciatore, cioppino, pasta marinara (no meat), shrimp marinara, shrimp primavera, stewed squid with tomatoes and peas, thin spaghetti with eggplant, thin spaghetti with red clam sauce, veal cacciatore

Desserts: fresh fruit whip, Italian ice, rice cake

Japanese:

Appetizers/Accompaniments: chicken and noodles in miso soup, chicken in grilled rice cake soup, clams and scallions in bean soup, miso soup, peas and rice, seafood sunomono, shrimp in rice cake soup, suimono, su-udon, sweet simmered Oriental vegetables, yaki-udon

Entrées: glaze-grilled scallops, nabemono, pinecone squid, pork and noodles in a soy-flavored broth, sashimi, shabu-shabu, sukiyaki (chicken or beef), sushi, teriyaki (chicken or seafood), yosenabe

Dessert: fresh fruit

Indian:

Appetizers/Accompaniments: aloo chole, biryani (shrimp or vegetable), chapati, chick-peas and spinach marinade, chutney (mint or onion), curried chick-peas, kulcha, lentils and spinach, naan, pulkas, pullao (plain, peas, or shrimp), onion salad, raita, rice pilaf with peas, rice with chick-peas, tamata salat, vegetable curry

Entrées: bhuna (fish or lamb), chicken tikka, kheema matter, lentils and vegetables with chicken or fish masala, rice and chicken pilaf, saag (chicken or lamb), tandoori chicken, vandaloo (beef, chicken, or fish)

Desserts: fruit salad with thickened milk, mango fool, pineapple fruit salad

Mexican:

Appetizers/Accompaniments: black bean soup, black beans, cantaloupe soup, ceviche, corn tortillas, gazpacho, "pot beans" (rather than refried beans), salsa, tortilla soup

Entrées: arroz con pollo, burrito (chicken or beef), camarones de hacha, fajitas (chicken or shrimp), shrimp enchilada, soft chicken taco (Note: For combination plates, choose only one entrée rather than the mucho grande entrée.)

Desserts: capirotada, flan

Middle Eastern:

Appetizers/Accompaniments: baba ghanoush, couscous, dolma, ful medames, hummus, lentil soup, miya dolma, pita bread, rice pilaf, tabouuli

Entrées: gyros, kibbeh, lah me june, sheik el mashi, shish kebab, souvlaki

Dessert: rice pudding

Thai:

Appetizers/Accompaniments: corn and shrimp soup, crystal noodle, pad jay, papaya and shrimp salad, pok taek, seafood kabob, shrimp and orange chili salad, squid salad, steamed mussels, steamed rice, sweet and sour cucumber, talay thong, tom yum koong, vegetable boat

Entrées: fried rice with chicken, garlic shrimp, poy sian, Thai chicken, seafood platter, scallops bamboo, sweet and sour chicken

Desserts: lychee nuts, mangoes and sticky rice, Thai fried banana

---

Note. From *The Restaurant Companion* by H. Warshaw, 1990, Chicago, IL: Surrey Books (800-326-4430). Adapted by permission of the publisher. Also from "The International Cuisines Calorie Counter" by Densie Webb. Copyright © 1990 by Densie Webb. Reprinted by permission of M. Evans & Co., Inc.

7

Surviving Fast Food Without Guilt

"I really don't like to eat fast food, but because of my daughter's gymnastic lessons, my son's soccer, my husband's meetings, and my full-time work schedule, it's often the best we can do for dinner."—

marketing manager

Take the *s* out of fast food and you get f-a-t food. If fat were helium, many people would float out of fast-food restaurants. Here are some examples of how a fast-food meal could quickly spell fat.

Meal	Calories	Fat (g)	% Fat calories
Burger King (breakfast) Bagel Sandwich, Hash Browns, Danish, Juice	1,421	84	53
Jack-in-the-Box Ultimate Cheeseburger, Onion Rings, Milk Shake	1,654	99	54
McDonald's McDLT, Large Fries, Milk Shake	1,300	61	42

Are you in fat shock? Don't worry. Eating fast food does not doom you to the valley of fat. But clearly, unless you choose carefully your diet easily could be swimming in fat.

Although most people downplay the extent to which they eat fast food (or they claim coercion by family or friends), the following statistics show that the fast-food industry is alive and well in the United States:

- Kentucky Fried Chicken served nearly *4.9 billion* pieces of chicken in 1989.
- 200 fast-food hamburgers are eaten per second.
- $60 billion was spent on fast food in 1989.

Most people do not consider eating at a fast-food restaurant to be dining out. It's more like stopping at a quick fueling station. Unfortunately, it's easy to tank up on the wrong kind of fuel for your body.

When you are in the "gulp-and-go" cycle, you may not give a second thought to what you put into your body. Furthermore, the portions don't seem so hefty, but a little food can add up quickly. For example, a relatively small biscuit sandwich with sausage and egg at McDonald's has a whopping 520 calories, and 60% of those calories are from fat.

DAMAGE CONTROL

Fortunately, you *can* eat at a fast-food place and fare relatively well. Almost every fast-food establishment has at least one healthy (or healthier) choice, which we'll consider later in this chapter. But first let's look at some hazards to avoid.

Beware of Healthy-Sounding Foods

Don't take anything for granted. Otherwise as you rush through your order, you may get plenty more than you intended. Table 7.1 gives some examples of fast foods which sound healthy but are actually loaded with fat.

Table 7.1   Healthy-Sounding Fatty Fast Foods

Food	Calories	% Fat calories
Arby's Chicken Cashew Salad	590	56
Burger King Chicken Sandwich	685	53
Carl's Jr. Bacon and Cheese Potato	730	53
Long John Silver's Seafood Platter	970	43
McDonald's Chef Salad with packet of Thousand Island Dressing	620	74
Taco Bell Taco Salad	905	61
Wendy's Chicken Club Sandwich	506	44

Those examples are rather depressing if you would have preferred to eat a hamburger all along—especially when you discover that a basic hamburger would be substantially lower in fat and calories! At least when you order french fries, you know what you are getting—fat—but that is a conscious choice.

Sometimes, foods that are not that high in fat content are still high in calories. El Pollo Loco, a growing West Coast fast-food subsidiary of Denny's, prides itself on using the American Heart Association guidelines to formulate most of its recipes (truly an honorable goal). Most people are surprised, then, to learn that the regular Combo meal has 720 calories! While these calories are not mainly from fat (33% fat calories), the caloric load is high for many people. These calories stack up due to the generous serving of three tortillas and because the skin is left on the chicken. In this case, my recommendation is split the meal and leave the skin off the chicken.

Mining for Fat Traps

Here are some guidelines to help keep your good intentions from going astray:

1. Anything fried is best avoided or limited. This includes the healthy-sounding alternatives, chicken and fish. Once these lower fat meats are fried, they are no better and can be even worse than a hamburger.

   For example, compare chicken nuggets versus a simple hamburger at McDonald's: Chicken McNuggets have 290 calories and 51% fat calories; a regular hamburger has 260 calories and significantly less fat, 33% fat calories. In this case, the hamburger is the better choice!

2. Be extra careful with salads. Greens would seem to be the obvious best choice, and they can be. The problem lies not in the salad, but in the dressing. Many salad dressing packages have at least 2 or more servings! For example, the dressings at McDonald's contain 4 to 5 servings. If you use the entire packet, you may be getting five times as many calories as you're expecting. Here are some fatty examples:

1 pkg Honey French Dressing (*Arby's*)	350 calories
1 pkg Olive Oil and Vinegar Dressing (*Burger King*)	310 calories
1 pkg Peppercorn Dressing (*McDonald's*)	400 calories

3. Potatoes at first glance would seem like a healthy choice in the burger world. But once crowned in cheese sauces, sour cream, chili, or bacon, the calories are easily doubled, and the fat level increased by 100-fold.
4. Hold the cheese. Although cheese is rich in calcium, it is loaded with saturated fat and cholesterol. Until the fast-food industry offers lowfat cheese, save your cheese-eating for home or grazing times when you have the lowfat varieties available.
5. If you must have a hamburger, go for the smallest version, generally a 2-1/2 to 3 ounce patty.
6. Avoid double trouble: double hamburgers, large fries.
7. Hold the goop (mayonnaise, special sauces, tartar sauce). Or, if the sauce is kept on, simply wipe it off with a napkin. The flavor will still be there, but most of the calories will be gone.

FAT CITY

If there were ever a most-wanted list for fatty food, many fast-food entrées would fit the bill. A large number of the foods these establishments offer contain over 55% fat calories. Granted, it's possible to balance out your fat and calorie budget for the day, but it can get mighty tough with some of these fast-food offerings. Some of the more notable fat assaults are listed in List 7.1.

SIDE ORDERS

The typical accompaniments to a fast-food meal, such as fries and a soda, can also do damage, so order carefully. There's nothing wrong

List 7.1
Among the Fattiest Fast Foods

These foods have at least 55% fat calories. (For exact fat counts, refer to Appendix B.)

Arby's

Breakfast: Sausage and Egg Croissant, Sausage Biscuit

Lunch/Dinner: Bac'n Cheddar Deluxe, Cherry Turnover, Chicken Cashew Salad, Philly Beef 'N Swiss, Steak Deluxe

Burger King

Breakfast: Biscuit with Sausage, Biscuit with Sausage and Egg, Croissan'wich (all varieties), Scrambled Egg Platter (all varieties), Danish

Lunch/Dinner: Bacon Double Deluxe Cheeseburger, Whopper (with Cheese, Double, Double with Cheese)

Carl's Jr.

Breakfast: Scrambled Eggs, Sunrise Sandwich with Sausage, Hashbrown Nuggets

Lunch/Dinner: Classic Double Cheeseburger, Double Western Bacon Cheeseburger, Famous Star Hamburger, Super Star Hamburger

Dairy Queen

Lunch/Dinner: Chicken Sandwich, DQ Hounder (all varieties), Hot Dog (with Chili or Cheese), Triple Hamburger, Triple Cheeseburger

Hardee's

Breakfast: Big Country Breakfast (with Sausage or Bacon), Biscuit sandwiches (Sausage; Sausage and Egg; Bacon, Egg, and Cheese), Hash Rounds

Lunch/Dinner: Bacon Cheeseburger

Jack-in-the-Box

Breakfast: Crescent (Supreme or Sausage), Hashbrowns

Lunch/Dinner: Bacon Cheeseburger, Chicken Supreme, Grilled Sourdough Burger, Ham and Turkey Melt, Super Taco, Taco Salad, Ultimate Cheeseburger

Kentucky Fried Chicken

Lunch/Dinner: Chicken Nuggets, Lite 'N Crispy (Thigh and Side Breast), all Original Recipe and Extra Tasty Crispy Fried Chicken Pieces (except center-cut breast)

Long John Silver's

Lunch/Dinner: Gumbo with Cod and Shrimp Bobs

McDonald's

Breakfast: Biscuit (with Sausage or Sausage and Egg), Scrambled Eggs, Sausage McMuffin with Egg

Lunch/Dinner: McDLT

Taco Bell

Lunch/Dinner: Mexican Pizza, Nachos Supreme, Taco Bellgrande, Taco Salad (with or without shell), Taco Supreme

Wendy's

Lunch/Dinner: Crispy Chicken Nuggets

with having french fries on occasion, but don't get into the habit of ordering them with your fast-food meal. To get an idea of how the side orders can top your calorie load, look at Table 7.2.

THE OTHER SIDE OF THE FAST-FOOD STORY

Now that you've learned about hidden fat traps and overt fat assaults in fast foods, take heart in knowing that there is nutrition value to be

Table 7.2   Basic Ranges for Side Orders

Side order	Calories	Fat (g)	% Fat calories	Sodium (mg)	Cholesterol (mg)
Cola and lemon-lime drinks					
12 oz	140	0	0	15	0
16 oz	190	0	0	20	0
22 oz	260	0	0	25	0
32 oz	380	0	0	40	0
French fries					
Small	200-221	10-12	45-49	110-164	8-10
Medium	320-353	17-20	48-51	150-262	12-21
Large	400-442	22-24	49-50	200-328	16
Onion rings	302-382	17-23	51-54	407-559	27
Salad dressing					
Regular	210-400	18-29	65-77	510-790	20-35
Reduced calorie	18-176	1-8	41-50	310-670	0

found in fast-food restaurants. Furthermore, it is easy to walk away with a healthier order. In almost every fast-food chain, it is possible to order a broiled chicken sandwich and/or a salad. This is progress! Some outlets also offer whole wheat bread and low-calorie salad dressing.

Fast-food chains continue to make changes to accommodate health-conscious customers. Taco Bell converted to corn oil rather than lard for their beans and tortillas. Most fast-food chains have converted to 100% vegetable shortening. (Reality check: Keep in mind, this only changes the *saturated* fat content, not the *total* fat content of a food. But it is a step in the right direction.) McDonald's now offers a fat-free muffin, and made healthy headlines when it introduced its McLean Deluxe sandwich—a hamburger considerably lower in fat. Kentucky Fried Chicken now offers Lite 'n Crispy chicken—chicken fried without the skin—an improvement, although the chicken still has significant fat levels. El Pollo Loco cooks chicken by broiling rather than frying. Take advantage of the healthier options that are now available.

BEST BETS FOR BUILDING A HEALTHY MEAL

Here's how you can order a meal in a fast-food restaurant without feeling guilty.

- Generally, you will be in better shape if you stick with the char-broiled or roasted sandwiches, especially chicken.
- Do go for the salads and salad bar. Just go easy on the dressings, as mentioned earlier.
- Try quenching your thirst with juice or lowfat milk. Diet sodas, coffee, and tea are also low-calorie options.
- Have a sweet tooth? Take advantage of the frozen yogurt offered in many fast-food places. An honorable mention goes to McDonald's here for their very lowfat shakes (less than 2 grams of fat in a shake).

Breakfast is also a challenge in fast-food restaurants. Basically, pass on the breakfast sandwiches, breakfast meats, fried potatoes, and eggs. Unlike conventional restaurants, French toast in a fast-food chain is usually deep-fried (more like a doughnut), so pass on that, too.

Instead choose pancakes, cold cereal, plain toast, or plain bagels. Apply margarine sparingly, if at all. Jam is a good fat-free alternative that is lower in calories than margarine.

Pizza can be a nutritious choice. Just stick with either plain cheese or a veggie. (Note: I recommend holding the olives—they have 97% fat calories.) Pass up the pepperoni and sausage. Be careful of deep-dish pizza. It's often dripping with oil because of a "greasy-pan policy." Some pizzerias load the pan with oil so that the pizza will slide right out.

To blot or not to blot? Does blotting your pizza with a napkin to soak up the excess oil pools from the melted cheese make a difference? To be honest, I don't know if it is a significant difference, but it has become a habit of mine! I figure every little bit helps, and it is easy to do.

To give you a healthy head start, Table 7.3 lists specific best bets by fast-food chain. (Lowfat milk and juice were not mentioned because of their obvious advantages.)

For nutritional information on other fast-food items, see Appendix B. Nutritional information on fast-food kid meals is in chapter 15.

Table 7.3   Best Bets in Fast Food

Fast food	Calories	Fat (g)	% Fat calories	Sodium (mg)	Cholesterol (mg)
Burger King:					
Bagel	272	6	20	438	29
Chunky Chicken Salad	142	4	25	443	49
Side Salad	25	0	0	25	0
Carl's Jr.:					
Blueberry Muffin	340	9	24	300	45
Bran Muffin	258	7	20	370	60
Charbroiler BBQ Chicken Sandwich	400	7	15	880	40
English Muffin with Margarine	190	5	24	280	0
Lite Potato	290	1	3	60	0
Domino's Pizza:					
2 Slices of Large (16-in.) Pie					
Cheese	376	10	24	483	19
Ham	417	11	24	805	26
El Pollo Loco:					
Beans*	110	1	12	450	n/a
Charbroiled Chicken Salad	200	4	16	375	65
Chicken Breast Sandwich	290	7	20	375	65
Corn	110	2	14	110	n/a
Corn Tortillas (3)	210	2	8	70	n/a

(Cont.)

Table 7.3   (Continued)

Fast food	Calories	Fat (g)	% Fat calories	Sodium (mg)	Cholesterol (mg)
Dole Whip	90	0	0	18	n/a
Rice	100	1	9	250	n/a
Hardee's:					
Chicken 'N Pasta Salad	230	3	12	380	55
Grilled Chicken Sandwich	310	9	26	890	60
Pancakes (3)	280	2	6	890	15
Regular Roast Beef	260	9	31	730	35
Jack-in-the-Box:					
Chicken Fajita Pita	292	8	25	703	34
Kentucky Fried Chicken:					
Corn-on-the-cob	176	3	15	21	1
Mashed Potatoes and Gravy	71	2	25	339	1
Long John Silver's:					
Baked Chicken	140	4	26	670	70
Baked Fish	120	1	8	120	110
Baked Fish with Lemon Breadcrumb Sprinkle	160	2	15	440	95
Baked Fish with Scampi Sauce	180	6	30	340	90
Bread Stick	110	3	25	120	0
Green Beans	30	trace	0	540	<5
Hushpuppy (1)	70	2	26	25	<5
Mixed Vegetables	60	2	30	330	0
Rice Pilaf	250	3	11	660	0
Seafood Salad	270	7	23	670	90
Side Salad	20	trace	0	20	0
McDonald's:					
Apple Bran Muffin	190	0	0	230	0
Cheerios	80	1	11	210	0
Chunky Chicken Salad	140	3	19	230	78
English Muffin with Butter	170	5	26	270	9
Hotcakes with Butter, Syrup	410	9	20	640	21
McLean Deluxe Sandwich	320	10	28	670	60
Wheaties	90	trace	0	220	0
Taco Bell:					
Bean Burrito (red sauce)	447	14	28	1,148	9

Fast food	Calories	Fat (g)	% Fat calories	Sodium (mg)	Cholesterol (mg)
Wendy's:					
Chili	220	7	29	750	45
Salad Bar**					
Breadsticks (2)	35	1	26	60	0
Pasta Salad (1/4 cup)	35	trace	0	120	n/a
Three Bean Salad (1/4 cup)	60	trace	0	15	n/a
Super Bar					
Alfredo Sauce (2 oz)	35	1	26	300	trace
Fettuccine (2 oz)	190	3	27	3	10
Flour Tortilla	110	3	25	220	n/a
Pasta Medley (2 oz)	60	2	30	5	trace
Picante Sauce (2 oz)	18	trace	0	5	n/a
Spaghetti Meat Sauce (2 oz)	60	2	30	315	10
Spaghetti Sauce (2 oz)	30	trace	0	345	trace
Spanish Rice (2 oz)	70	1	13	440	trace
Rotini (2 oz)	90	2	20	trace	trace

It is best to hold the margarine or butter, even though some items include it.

n/a = data not available.

*Although El Pollo Loco beans have lard, the amount of fat is very small (1 g).

**At Wendy's Salad Bar, remember fresh fruits and produce are always Best Bets.

8

Deli Dos and Don'ts

Dashing through a deli is a popular way to fend for yourself at mealtime. But if you like it piled high, you could be in for some deep fatty surprises.

Take a quick look at some examples of how easily you can fall prey to deli cuisine—even the healthy-sounding sandwiches. Here's an example from Subway:

Sandwich	Calories	Fat (g)	% Fat calories
Seafood and Lobster (foot-long)	974	54	50
Tuna on wheat (foot-long)	1,132	73	58

DELI DON'Ts

Let's look at the nutritional dark side of deli sandwiches first, so you can maneuver around the fat traps. Here are some offenders that can do you in on standard deli orders:

1. Large sandwiches (even a small is big).
2. Globs of mayonnaise (due in part to the larger surface area from the bread roll and the industrial-size spatulas they are painted on with).
3. Numerous fatty meats and cheeses. The quantity of meat is usually between 4 to 6 ounces. Compare how just the type of filling you select can make a big fat difference in Table 8.1.

Table 8.1   Deli Meats Comparison

Each of the following is based on a 4-oz portion:

Deli meat	Calories	Fat (g)	% Fat calories	Cholesterol (mg)
Bologna, beef	351	32	82	63
Bologna, turkey	232	18	71	76
Ham, regular (11% fat)	208	12	52	n/a
Ham, turkey	143	6	35	67
Mortadella	350	28	73	60
Pastrami, beef	396	33	75	104
Pastrami, turkey	132	5	33	58
Salami, beef and pork	278	22	73	73
Salami, turkey	200	14	61	80
Sausage, Polish	368	32	79	80
Sausage, turkey	208	14	61	88
Turkey breast	123	2	12	48

n/a = data not available.

Note. From *Bowes & Church's Food Values of Portions Commonly Used* (15th ed.) by J.A.T. Pennington, 1989, Philadelphia, PA: J.B. Lippincott Co. Adapted by permission of the publisher.

4. Beware of fatty surprises lurking in vegetarian sandwiches, such as cheese, avocado, chopped olives, and more cheese! All of these ingredients are fatty.

   To give you a glimpse of how easily calories and fat pile up (if you are not careful), look at Table 8.2 for nutritional values of deli sandwiches.
5. Many delis have salads that might be the equivalent of a sandwich, except the meat is on a bed of lettuce without the roll. Surprisingly, salads can be particularly high in fat because of dressings, mayonnaise, cheese, and meats. For example, these

large salads from Subway are high in fat and calories even before salad dressing is added:

Salad	Calories	Fat (g)	% Fat calories	Cholesterol (mg)
Seafood and Crab	639	54	75	56
Seafood and Lobster	597	49	75	55
Tuna	756	68	81	85

And still more fat: Remember, this data does not include dressing, which could easily add up to an extra 300 calories!

Table 8.2   Deli Sandwiches: Calories, Fat, and Cholesterol

Nutritional data for most delis are either nonexistent or unavailable to the public. One exception is Subway. They have generously provided their nutritional information. The data listed below are based on foot-long whole wheat rolls.

Subway sandwich	Calories	Fat (g)	% Fat calories	Cholesterol (mg)
BMT (bologna, genoa, ham, cheese, and pepperoni)	1,011	57	50	133
Club (roast beef, ham, cheese, and turkey breast)	722	23	29	84
Cold Cut Combo (turkey bologna, turkey ham, cheese, and turkey salami)	883	41	42	166
Ham and Cheese	673	22	30	73
Meatball (with cheese)	947	45	43	88
Roast Beef	716	24	30	75
Seafood and Crab (with cheese)	1,015	58	52	56
Seafood and Lobster	974	54	50	55
Spicy Italian (salami, pepperoni, and cheese)	1,073	64	54	137
Steak and Cheese	711	33	41	82
Tuna (with cheese)	1,132	73	58	85
Turkey Breast (with cheese)	673	20	27	67
Veggies and Cheese	565	18	29	n/a

n/a = data not available.

DELI DOs

It's becoming much easier to make lighter selections. In fact, one chain, Blimpies, made national news when it introduced its light menu with sandwiches under 300 calories. Bravo. Look at Table 8.3 for some best bets in deli sandwiches.

Table 8.3   Best Bets in Deli Sandwiches

Here are some good deli choices, based on data supplied by Subway and Blimpies.

Sandwich	Calories	Fat (g)	% Fat calories	Cholesterol (mg)
Blimpies:				
Ham Swiss Pita	276	8	25	58
Ham Turkey Swiss Pita	226	5	21	36
Seafood/Crab Pita	199	0	0	35
Turkey Pita	193	5	23	13
Subway*:				
6-in. Ham and Cheese	337	11	30	37
6-in. Roast Beef	358	12	30	38
6-in. Subway Club	361	12	29	42
6-in. Turkey Breast	337	10	27	34
6-in. Veggies and Cheese	282	9	29	n/a

n/a = data not available.

*If you hold the cheese and oil, you will save additional calories. Or if you can use the extra calories, the foot-long versions of these sandwiches would be acceptable (but double the calories).

Fortunately, delis are used to custom making your sandwiches. Here are some suggestions.

1. Order the smallest sandwich, generally the half sandwich or the small. You will still get ample food. (It just might seem smaller next to a foot-long sandwich.)
2. Hold the mayo. Extra tip: Be sure to make this request even if you are ordering a mayonnaise-based salad sandwich such as tuna. Many places will still put additional mayo on the bread!
3. For fat-free tasty spreads, request one of the following: vinegar (this tastes surprisingly good), diet Italian dressing, or mustard.

4. If in a grocery store deli, ask them to weigh your meat and limit it to 3 ounces.
5. Have meats sliced extra thin. It piles nice and high, giving you the illusion of more.
6. Request extra lettuce, tomatoes, and onions.
7. Choose the leanest cuts of meat (this can make a tremendous difference).
8. Hold the chips. (Even if they are free, ask that they not be included with your sandwich. Why tempt yourself?)
9. Beans and garden salads make good side dish choices. Pass on goopy salads such as coleslaw, macaroni salad, and potato salad.
10. Request a whole wheat roll or bread.
11. Hold the cheese unless lowfat varieties are available.
12. Hold the oil. Many sub sandwich places automatically squirt oil on the bread before adding the filling.

9

Satisfying the Sweet Tooth

"I would usually have frozen yogurt for lunch."—
busy secretary

Be it a snack attack or pseudomeal, sweet tooths and munchies can strike at any time, especially when you are on the run. The first line of defense is to remember the golden rule: Go no longer than 5 hours without eating. You are most vulnerable when you are hungry, so following this rule can help prevent minibinges.

It can be very easy to give in to an ''urge to splurge.'' There seem to be unlimited opportunities: mall food courts, bakeries, corner doughnut shops, and ice-cream and yogurt shops. Generally if your weight and blood cholesterol are in good control, occasional splurges will not get you into trouble. It is what you eat on a consistent basis that counts.

MAKING THE MOST OF SNACK ATTACKS

First, here are some general guidelines:

- Keep it small. Most snack shops have child-size portions or small servings available.

- If you don't love it, don't eat it. When it comes to eating fun foods, most of us don't have a lot of extra calories to play around with. Every bite counts. That's why if you happen to eat a goodie just because it's there, chances are you will not satisfy your underlying goody tooth. Before you know it, you will be on the prowl again.
- Savor. I believe that part of the reason people keep coming back for more treats is they did not let themselves experience the pleasure the first time around. If you are feeling guilty, you truly are not enjoying the food moment. Patients have told me that they knew what they were doing was ''wrong.'' So although they continued to eat, they did so at a quick pace, pseudodenial style. Sit down and experience what you are eating.
- Don't make goodies a routine habit, and don't let them become associated with certain activities. It could haunt you. For example, don't become ''obligated'' to buy an ice-cream cone every time you are in the mall, or you will train your body to expect the indulgence every time you shop.

Chill Thrills: Frozen Yogurt

Thanks to the proliferation of frozen yogurt, it is possible to quell a sweet tooth without getting into a diet crisis.

For example, Penguins Fat-Free Frozen Yogurt has 0 grams of fat and only 20 calories per ounce. Most fat-free frozen yogurts are comparable and range between 20 to 25 calories per ounce.

If you go to the trouble of having a fat-free dessert, don't drown it in fatty toppings. Consider what these toppings may be adding:

Topping	Calories	Fat (g)	% Fat calories
1/4 cup chocolate chips	228	13	49
1/4 cup peanut butter chips	228	13	51
1/3 cup hot fudge	248	10	36

Best Bets. Stick with the fat-free frozen yogurts and, of course, watch those toppings. I suggest you have it in a regular cone because you tend to eat it slower and are less likely to be tempted by troublesome toppings. Of course, fresh fruit toppings are no problem. Frozen yogurt shops such as TCBY, Heidi's, and Penguins all offer a large selection of nonfat frozen yogurts. Many fast-food chains also offer frozen yogurt.

Ice Cream

If you prefer the density and texture of ice cream, there are some lower fat options that taste great. One ice-cream shop, Lappert's, has a delicious line of fat-free ice creams. Baskin-Robbins, famous for its rich 31 flavors, also has a variety of lower fat ice creams.

If you are fond of the traditional ice-cream desserts, the selected data in Table 9.1 illustrate how easy it is to slide down the calories at Baskin-Robbins and Dairy Queen.

Best Bets.   Go for the lowfat or fat-free ice creams. Sorbets, fruit ices, and frozen fruit whips are also good no-fat choices. Remember, though, fat-free does not mean calorie-free. If you must have that sundae, choose the smallest size and hold the whip cream. Most ice-cream shops now also have frozen yogurts.

Table 9.1   Ice-Cream Treats

Treat	Calories	Fat (g)	% Fat calories
Baskin-Robbins:			
1 regular scoop ice cream			
Chocolate Raspberry Truffle	310	17	49
Daiquiri Ice	140	0	0
Rainbow Sherbet	160	2	11
Vanilla	240	14	53
World Class Chocolate	280	14	45
Light Ice Cream (1/2 cup)	110-130	3-6	25-42
Fat Free	100	0	0
Sugar Free (1/2 cup)	80-100	1-2	11-18
Sorbet Fruit Whip (4 oz)	80	0	0
Dairy Queen:			
Banana Split	540	11	18
Cone, small	140	4	26
Cone, large	340	10	26
Chocolate Dipped Cone, small	190	9	43
Chocolate Dipped Cone, large	510	24	42
Float	410	7	15
Hot Fudge Brownie Delight	600	20	30
Sundae, small	190	4	19
Sundae, large	440	10	20

Honorable Mention: McDonald's milk shakes are a very lowfat treat with a maximum of 2 grams of fat per shake. Just beware that although the fat content is low, one shake has about 290 to 320 calories. This still fares much better than a typical milk shake. Compare the difference:

Milk shake	Calories	Fat (g)	% Fat calories
Dairy Queen Shake	490-990	13-26	24
McDonald's Milk Shake	290-320	1-2	3-5

Cinnamon Rolls

My daughter is mesmerized by watching cinnamon rolls made by hand. Just the smell of cinnamon can drive even the staunchest health-conscious type to a slow drool.

Best Bets.   Think small and hold the extra icing. All too often, cinnamon pastries are made ultragiant size. Table 9.2 illustrates the difference with data courtesy of T.J. Cinnamon's. The petite size is your better bet, rather than the mini. Surprised? This is because the minis are not sold individually, but in fives called a "cinnacone." In this form, you are getting the second most caloric and the fattiest order!

Cookies

The aroma of fresh-baked cookies can arouse the cookie monster in all of us. But when the cookie crumbles into your mouth, the calorie and fat totals grow. Butter is usually a prime contributor to the fat attack, but little goodies such as chocolate chips, nuts, and coconut all add to the fat load.

Unfortunately, nutritional data from fresh cookie makers is limited. One of my most frustrating experiences was trying to get nutritional data on Mrs. Fields' self-proclaimed "cholesterol free" cookies. If a company is making a nutritional claim they should be obligated to back it up with nutrition facts. I called several times and was not able to get any nutritional information. Later, I spoke to one of Debbie Fields' assistants only to receive the following note in the mail, signed by Debbie Fields:

Dear Cookie Lover,

Thanks for your interest in Mrs. Fields' Cookies. I'm sorry, I haven't a clue as to the calorie count of my cookies, nor do I have nutritional information.

Mrs. Fields' Cookies are made with only the finest ingredients such as: real creamery butter, pure vanilla, and a special blend of chocolate formulated especially for the Mrs. Fields' Cookie Company.

My most recent phone attempts (many months later) have only revealed that Mrs. Fields plans to provide nutritional information, but not for several months. (It only takes a few minutes to analyze a recipe.)

Table 9.2, however, provides a cookie data comparison from three fast-food companies and Famous Amos (which is phasing out its fresh cookie stands).

Best Bets.   Go for the tiny treats (about the size of a quarter). That way, you appease your taste buds without the typical calorie load. Oatmeal cookies are a better bite, but don't kid yourself—they also carry a fat burden.

Table 9.2   Baked Treats

Treat	Calories	Fat (g)	% Fat calories
T.J. Cinnamon's Cinnamon Rolls:			
Cinnacone (5 mini)	375	25	60
Junior	235	13	50
Mini	75	5	60
Petite	185	10	49
Original Gourmet	630	34	49
Cookies:			
Carl's Jr. Chocolate Chip Cookie	353	16	41
Famous Amos Chocolate Chip with Pecans (tiny size: 8 g)	40	2	47
Hardee's Big Cookie	250	13	47
McDonald's Chocolaty Chip Cookies (1 pkg)	330	16	43

10

Meals to Fly High On

"I travel all the time—it's hard for me to eat right."—
C.E.O. of national company

Logging frequent-flyer miles doesn't mean an end to your health. But sometimes long trips, or unexpected delays that leave you stranded in an airport, can make you vulnerable not only to jet lag but also to meal drag.

AIRPORT TRAPS

This chapter will show you how to make the best of air travel. Let's start first with the airport itself.

Missed Planes and Missed Meals

A delayed plane can mean a delayed or missed meal. While waiting for your plane, you may find that familiar foods with recognizable brand names can be quite appealing—especially when you are new in a city. It is no wonder that specialty food stores such as Häagen-Dazs seem to do brisk business in an airport.

Don't let your guard down just because you are traveling. Comfort foods and novel delicacies will tempt you when traveling. Indulging in treats on occasion is no problem. But if you are a regular flyer, frequent treats can be trouble.

Eating in airports is similar to eating out, so the restaurant tips discussed in chapter 6 apply here as well. Just recognize that you're likely to eat out of boredom when you're in an airport.

Be sure to pack some survival snacks for unexpected delays. There's nothing worse than being stranded at an airport with the food stands closed, while dinner is flying high without you. Light-weight but nutritious snacks include miniboxes of raisins, whole grain crackers, and miniboxes of cereal.

Killing Time—Not Your Diet

For some weary travelers, eating might seem to be the most exciting thing to do in the airport. If this sounds like you, you could be headed for diet distress (gourmet candy shops, ice-cream shops, cookie outlets). Snack attacks on fatty comfort foods can be trouble, and airports can magnify the damage. For example, I know of a person who always feels compelled to buy a one-pound box of Fannie May chocolates during a layover (these are usually eaten by arrival time). When you consider that one pound of Hershey's chocolate Kisses has 2,460 calories, you can imagine the fat and calorie content of rich chocolates such as Fannie May.

"Lounging around" in the airport lounge can also inflict serious damage to your diet. Sipping cocktails and munching on free appetizers until your plane comes in can severely burden your calorie tab. And did you know many of those free appetizers are high in salt and are set out with the intention of making you thirsty so you'll purchase more beverages? That means even more calories. Don't fall into this trap.

Strategies

Plan ahead. Bring along extra reading material (or even some work to do). Some airports offer amenities such as on-site health clubs and barber/beauty shops. Take advantage of them. The best 2 hours I ever spent in an airport were in Dallas—where I treated myself to a massage and a manicure!

IN-FLIGHT MEALS

One of the best tips I received for airline meals was from a patient who was a seasoned commercial pilot. His advice: Order the special meals. Ironically, his reason was not health; he found the taste to be consistently superior!

I too have found special meals to be very tasty. Once, a passenger sitting beside me wanted to know if I was flying first class. He thought this because of the special meal I received. In this case, it was the fresh seafood platter with jumbo shrimp and real crab!

Special meals vary considerably depending on the airline carrier, but they tend to fall into three classes:

- Religious—Kosher, Hindu, Moslem
- Special Diet—diabetic, low-cholesterol, low-sodium
- Other—light, heart-healthy, seafood platter, vegetarian

In most cases, ordering a special meal is simply a phone call away. You can do it when you make your plane reservations. Most airlines require 6 to 24 hours' notice. United Airlines changed their policy in 1990 and now requires only 6 hours' advance notice. And you can't beat the price of special meals: no extra charge.

By ordering special meals, you also help influence what's served. According to a November 1990 *Newsweek* report, special meal requests nearly doubled in the past few years and triggered a new healthy impetus in traditional coach menus.

If you are unable to order a special meal, an important eating lesson can be learned from regular airline meals. Note the portion size of the meat (usually chicken or beef)—it is usually about 3 to 4 ounces.

Fly High Surprises

Although portions for standard airline meals are small, don't let that fool you. According to the dietitian who works for Sky Chefs, an airline caterer that prepares 50,000 meals daily for several airlines, a typical coach meal can easily run over 600 calories.

Ironically, I have worked with a number of people who regard their in-flight meal as only a snack. These misguided souls proceed to have a "real meal" when they arrive at their destination. That's how you get into calorie traps.

Examples of how the calories can quickly stack up are listed in Table 10.1, courtesy of Sky Chefs' dietitian. Note, the meals do not include the beverage calories. You can see that a typical airline meal is certainly no snack when it comes to calories and fat.

Table 10.1   In-Flight Meals: The Calories Can Fly High

This data is from actual meals served in coach class.

Meal	Calories	Fat (g)	% Fat calories
Roasted Chicken Meal: Roasted chicken (skinless), rice pilaf, green beans, green salad with vinegar and oil dressing, 2 slices whole wheat bread, 1 pat margarine, shortbread cookies **Total:**	738	34	41
Beef Burgundy Meal: Beef ribs, rice pilaf, green beans, green salad with vinegar and oil dressing, 2 slices whole wheat bread, 1 pat margarine, shortbread cookies **Total:**	836	51	55
Lasagna Meal: Lasagna, green salad with vinegar and oil dressing, Parmesan cheese, sesame crackers, 1 pat margarine, cookies **Total:**	778	52	60
Chef's Salad Plate: Chef's salad, ranch-style dressing, whole wheat roll, 1 pat margarine, croutons, cookies **Total:**	610	41	60
Grilled Chicken Sandwich: Chicken sandwich, green salad with vinegar and oil dressing, whole wheat roll, 1 pat margarine, cookies **Total:**	928	62	60
Snack: 1 small bag of peanuts	166	14	76

Data courtesy of Sky Chefs.

Health-conscious travelers can make airline meals lighter by making a few small changes. If you omit the margarine and use only half a packet of salad dressing, that would save about 70 calories. If you skip dessert, that would be another 155 calories saved.

Lighten Your Load

Here are more ideas to lighten your traveling load:

1. Get in the habit of reserving a special meal when you make your plane reservations.

2. Skip the nuts. I don't know why nuts are the most common snack served, but if you are watching your waistline or fat intake, you'll want to pass on these. Nuts can be anywhere from 69% to 93% fat calories.

3. Drink a glass of water or juice for every hour in flight. The American Dietetic Association recommends this to help minimize jet lag and prevent dehydration.

Special tasty tip: Request half orange juice with mineral water or club soda for a refreshing drink. This combination also hides the tin flavor of canned orange juice.

Alcoholic beverages are best avoided because they can aggravate water loss. Alcohol is a diuretic; it causes the body to lose water. And alcohol is second only to fat in its calorie content—ounce for ounce alcohol has nearly twice the calories of carbohydrates or protein.

4. If you don't have a special meal, minimize the use of added fat such as margarine and salad dressings. Remove skin from chicken. Pass on the dessert. An easy way to remove "sweet temptation" is to offer it to your fellow passenger. Or request it be left off your tray.

5. At breakfast, pass on the eggs and sausage (a typical hot meal). Instead get cold cereal, which usually comes with fresh fruit and a choice of lowfat or nonfat milk.

6. If you are scheduled for a lunch or dinner meeting when your plane arrives, either request the *special* fruit plate or pass on the meal. (Eating double meals can easily ground your healthy intentions.)

7. Be sure to check your itinerary for meal service. Never assume a meal will be served. Sometimes due to time zone changes the airline meal schedule may not match your stomach schedule. Plan ahead, or you may be desperately gobbling down peanut bags (at 166 calories a pop).

SPECIFIC AIRLINE OFFERINGS

Airline carriers were willing to share what types of special meals they offer, but they did not usually have specific nutritional information available. Here are the types of meals you can get from different airline carriers.

Alaska Airlines.   Alaska Airlines takes their food very seriously. The executives are required to eat the coach-class entrées two times weekly. These are the types of meals available:

Special Diet:	Bland, diabetic, low-cholesterol, low-sodium, and low-calorie
Religious:	Kosher
Other:	Strict vegetarian, lacto-ovo vegetarian, fruit plate, seafood, and child

American Airlines.   This is one of the few airlines that had some (limited) nutritional information on their special meals. They are working on a more detailed nutritional analysis of their special meals.

American also offers a unique approach to healthier meal service, called American Traveler, which was constructed in conjunction with the guidelines of the American Heart Association and the Cooper Clinic to provide heart-healthy meals. Here's what American Airlines offers:

Meal		Calories	Fat (g)	% Fat calories
Special Meals:	Low-cholesterol	400	10	23
	Low-calorie	425	n/a	n/a
	Diabetic	425	n/a	n/a
	American Traveler	500	18	32

Other meals available include Kosher, vegetarian, bland/soft, and low-sodium (118 mg of sodium). Data was not available for these meals.

Continental.   According to Siegfried Lang, manager of food and beverage planning, Continental is working on many projects to make their inflight offerings more healthy including:

- grilling most meat items, especially chicken,
- upgrading vegetarian entrées,
- offering a variety of freshly grilled fish with lowfat accompaniments, such as a cucumber-dill salsa, and
- developing a city-by-city tracking system to monitor the number of special meals served.

The company offers the following meal types:

Special Diet:	Diabetic, low-cholesterol, low-fat, and low-sodium
Religious:	Kosher, Hindu, and Moslem

Other: Fruit plate, infant, and child

Delta Air Lines. Delta has been working on providing healthier meals to its passengers. Here are a few changes they have implemented recently:

- Replaced sweet rolls and filled croissants with healthy types of muffins such as bran or multigrain
- Removed skin from baked chicken
- Eliminated products with tropical oils
- Added new menu items including grilled chicken, whole wheat rolls, and whole grain breads

These are the meals offered by Delta:

Special Diet: Bland, diabetic, low-calorie, low-cholesterol, lowfat, and low-sodium
Religious: Kosher, Hindu, and Moslem
Other: Pure vegetarian, ovo-lacto vegetarian, fruit plate, seafood, baby, toddler, and child

Pan Am. Pan Am is trying to alter their menu to reflect the consumer's interest in healthy eating, according to a company spokesperson. Advance notice of 8 hours is required to order special meals.
    Gourmet meals (nine different entrées) are available to anyone who joins the frequent-flyer program, World Pass. (Note that gourmet does not necessarily mean healthy.) The following meals are provided for domestic flights:

Special Diet: Low-sodium, lowfat, low-calorie, low-cholesterol, diabetic, bland, soft, and gluten-free
Religious: Moslem, Kosher, Hindu-vegetarian, and Hindu-nonvegetarian
Other: Children's, vegetarian, hot seafood, cold seafood, birthday cakes, wedding cakes, and World Pass gourmet meals (need 24 hours' advance notice)

United Airlines. United serves an average of 6,000 special meals per day (about 3% of their meals). The average meat entrée is between 3 and 4 ounces. They have added more chicken (skinless) and pasta due to consumer demand. United's in-flight dining director says their average meal has 400 calories and all their special diet meals are under 300 calories. United offers the following meals:

Special Diet: Diabetic, low-calorie, low-cholesterol, and low-sodium

Religious: Kosher, Hindu, and Moslem

Other: Traveler's light choice, seafood plate, fruit plate, and vegetarian

U.S. Air. U.S. Air is currently revamping all their menus to reflect consumer health trends. "We are going much lighter across the board," says Judy Silva, manager of menu planning and design. They offer only broiled chicken and have eliminated most sauces that were not light. They increase fiber at every opportunity; they use sprouted wheat bread in their french toast and whole grains in all bread categories; and they have increased the quantity of fresh fruits and vegetables. In addition, they lightened up their regular menu by providing light syrup and light cream cheese on a routine basis. The following meal types are offered by U.S. Air:

Special Diet: Diabetic, low-sodium, low-cholesterol, lowfat, and low-calorie

Religious: Kosher

Other: Child and vegetarian

11

Occupational
Eating Hazards

**"I don't have time for lunch. If I am lucky, I can sneak
a snack between clients."**—

financial advisor

Power meals and cutting deals, meetings drowning in doughnuts,
and doing business on the road are examples of occupational eating
hazards. This chapter will give you some quick tips to navigate
around risky eating conditions that can be found in any job.

MEETINGS AND DOUGHNUTS EVERYWHERE

Remember my motto, "Breakfast—don't leave home without it." It
needn't be a big meal; a light morning snack will help keep you out
of trouble. On an empty stomach, anything goes, and that can easily
be an unintended doughnut.

Strategy

If you can, find out who orders the doughnuts where you work and
suggest bagels and fresh fruit instead of, or at least in addition to,

the sweets. Most bakeries that supply doughnuts have no problem providing bagels. Another fat-free but tasty option: fat-free pastries (they are a superior alternative to Danish and doughnuts, but they will have an ample supply of sugar).

Even if you're able to steer clear of the doughnuts, you're still not out of danger. Coffee guzzling can be double trouble. First, most workplaces have a pot of coffee brewing all day long. It's very easy to slowly sip 1 cup an hour, or 8 to 10 cups of coffee a day. This is quite a caffeine load. Plus, if you are throwing in sugar or cream, you are giving yourself a double whammy of up to 400 to 500 extra calories.

There's also a caveat here. What does your cup of coffee look like (size-wise)? Styrofoam cups average about 6 ounces (3/4 cup). If you use a coffee mug, as many people do, you are probably drinking 12 ounces or 1-1/2 cups of coffee.

Let me illustrate how significant these calories can be. I had a client who worked as a private nurse. She came to me because she was frustrated at her inability to lose weight. I asked her the routine questions, including her coffee drinking habits—which added up to about 16 ounces six to eight times a day, with creamer! She was unknowingly drinking about 300 to 400 extra calories a day. She was able to lose weight primarily by simply cutting down her coffee intake and eliminating the nondairy creamer.

Strategy

Limit regular coffee to no more than 12 ounces. Rather than nondairy creamers, try nonfat powdered milk or, for convenience, the Weight Watchers Dairy Creamer packets. Or keep nonfat milk in the office refrigerator. Of course, drinking coffee black will cut out the calories completely.

POWER MEALS AND CUTTING DEALS

Let's face it, the goal of power meals is not power eating, but rather making a connection or cutting a deal. This is all the more reason to keep your food very simple. Focus your energies on the conversation, not on what you are eating. Now is not the time to make a fatty splurge on a meal that you are not likely to savor. Reserve your occasional feasts and special treats to times that you can relish them.

Strategy

Stick with simple, easy-to-eat foods. Who wants spaghetti on their face or alfalfa sprouts hanging out of their teeth when trying to make an impression? Refer back to chapter 6 on how to innocuously order a healthy meal without getting into a dog-and-pony show—especially if wining and dining are regular components of your job.

Simple entrées such as lemon chicken or broiled fresh fish make for an easy-to-handle meal that won't overload your fat budget.

VENDING MACHINE ROULETTE

Many of us have played this game. It's late afternoon, your stomach starts to churn, and you turn to the vending machines. Your traditional choices are often between candy bars and chips. Although small in size, these little guys are doing more than tiding you over:

Item	Calories	Fat (g)	% Fat calories
Kit Kat	244	13	48
Kudos Bar	170-200	9-12	48-57
Potato chips	148	10	61
Reese's Peanut Butter Cups (2)	281	17	54
Snickers Bar (king-size)	510	24	42

Strategy

Pretzels are a good lowfat choice—a one-ounce bag has only 111 calories. Try talking to the person responsible for the vending machine contracts and see if it is possible to include other options such as fresh fruit, juice, pop-top tuna, and cereal.

CATERING TRUCKS

My clients fondly call these traveling food establishments ''roach coaches.'' In spite of this, they continue to frequent them. The familiar horn blows, and workers flock to these at-your-door food venues. The problem here is most foods are already prepared and wrapped to go; it's like a movable vending machine.

Strategy

If you are a "regular," make requests for the next day (so your needs can be fulfilled at the master kitchen). For example, request a turkey sandwich to be prepared without cheese and mayonnaise. If your vending truck operator is not flexible, you will be better off bringing your own food. But here are some best bets commonly available: nonfat yogurt, plain bagels, juice, and nonfat or lowfat milk.

UNPREDICTABLE SCHEDULES AND EATING INTERRUPTUS

Thanks to car phones and beepers, the end to a well-planned schedule is only a beep away. You are often at the mercy of the caller. But this need not be a food disaster.

Physicians, fire fighters, and others who at a moment's notice are off to avert a crisis are especially vulnerable. Sales representatives, quality assurance people, and those in management jobs also are easily called away to solve a problem. This may make eating seem impossible.

Strategy

Remember, do not go longer than 5 hours without eating. If you are subject to frequent eating interruptus, you would do best to keep a stash of grazing snacks in your work environment (review chapter 2). Take advantage of the office kitchen, which exists in many settings. Keep it well stocked for unexpected "fire fighting." Keep healthy frozen meals stocked in the freezer.

ON THE ROAD AGAIN

Sales representatives, truckers, and others who spend time on the road daily are subject to eating pitfalls. Fast food quickly gets boring, and time to actually sit down in a coffee-shop type of restaurant is a rare luxury. Some people opt for a shorter lunch to wind up the day quicker.

Strategy

Keep a portable cooler stocked with easy grazing snacks and beverages. Consider packing some one-minute meals (see chapter 18).

OFFICE POLITICS: EATING YOUR WAY UP THE CORPORATE LADDER

You may be working very hard to impress your superiors in order to climb your way to the top. You must perform above and beyond the call of duty and never let your guard down. That advice also applies to eating.

Executive Dining Room

Eating in the executive dining room is not only a perk but an opportunity to network with key people in the company. Unfortunately, executive dining privileges are not immune from fatty foods.

Strategy

If possible ask the chef to prepare your foods without the customary butters and sauces. If your company has an on-site wellness program, suggest the dining service work with it by offering at least one health-smart entrée. Eating-out strategies from chapter 6 also will work here.

Long Hours

Whether you are doing time to build your corporate résumé or are just chronically overworked (by choice or demand), spending long hours on the job can do you in nutritionally if you are not prepared. Under these conditions it is easy to go longer than 5 hours without eating. For example, you eat lunch at noon and don't get off until six.

At other times you are so bombarded with work that you literally don't have time to think about food.

Attitude Adjustment: Consider food necessary for survival of the corporate fittest. How can you be doing your best work when you are running on empty? Remember, you can trick your body into thinking it's not hungry, but you will eventually pay the price.

Strategy

On the days when you know you will put in the ultrahours, plan ahead and stock your desk, briefcase, or company refrigerator with energizing grazing snacks. Or pack a double lunch.

For unexpected late hours, take a food break. If time is so precious that you can't even make it over to a fast-food place (healthy choices, of course), have a pizza delivered. Domino's, famous for its timely delivery service, has only 24% fat calories in its cheese pizza. Having a brief pizza party will also be a good morale booster, which could enhance productivity.

Office Potlucks and Birthday Parties

Nothing beats the lunch-box blues like an office potluck or birthday party. And the eating pressure is on. I'm not sure which is worse, a well-meaning relative trying to cram a specialty food down your throat or a co-worker or boss gently coercing you to "try it."

Strategy

First, set a good example by bringing something delicious and healthy. Second, control what you are eating by taking taster-size portions, the same strategy as with buffet dining. Last and very important, immediately throw away your plate when you are finished. This will make you less tempted to have unnecessary seconds and will keep overbearing colleagues from forcing more food on you.

Food Gifts

"Good job," says a boss, and gives you a box of gourmet chocolates. Or an appreciative client sends you a tin of cookies. Obviously, you do not want to shun good intentions, but if you bring the goodies home, you will be in for nonstop temptation.

Strategy

Fortunately, the solution is very easy. Share the "wealth" and calories. An occasional treat will not be a health disaster for you or your colleagues. But don't pressure your colleagues into eating something they don't want or need either. A local food bank will be most accepting of any food offering.

Desktop Goody Jars

These are time wasters and fat traps. One bitsy candy here, and another on the way back. Harmless? No. It's a good example of how eating amnesia works. Goody jars will often invite more people into your work space, which might be fun but can also become a nuisance and an unwanted distraction. And refills get expensive.

Strategy

Get rid of the desktop goody jars.

Giving at the Office

Girl Scout cookies, Little League candy bars . . . It seems as if there is always a time when a colleague (or boss) is helping their kid out by selling goodies for a fund-raiser.

Strategy

Go ahead and give a donation if you feel inclined, but decline the candy bar. Otherwise, you know what will invariably happen around midafternoon. Don't put yourself through that temptation. Since the real purpose of selling the treats is to raise money, giving money without receiving the goods will not be in bad taste.

Happy Hour

This after-work time can be a fun way to get to know colleagues in a relaxed atmosphere. But the alcoholic beverages with the accompanying appetizers can send you into calorie heaven. Table 11.1 gives some eye-opening examples.

Strategy

Get into the habit of ordering mineral water with a twist. Remember the purpose of happy hour is to network and socialize with co-workers. If you do drink alcohol, stick with the simpler beverages such as wine (which averages about 100 calories per glass). You may want to try

Table 11.1   Happy Hour Worries

Drink	Calories
Gin and tonic (7.5 oz)	171
Martini (2.5 oz)	156
Piña colada (4.5 oz)	262
Screwdriver (7 oz)	174

Appetizer	Calories
Cocktail meatballs	157
Crunch party mix (1 serving)	202
Nachos (1 serving)	308
Nut mix (1/4 cup)	219
Sweet and sour franks	132

the ''every other method,'' in which you drink a noncaloric beverage such as club soda after each alcoholic drink. This can cut your alcohol consumption (and its calories) in half.

Limit the appetizers as well. Here are some best bets: popcorn, chicken mini-tacos, pretzels, oysters, shrimp, and crab. Hold the chips, buffalo wings, meatballs, franks, dips, cheeses, and potato skins.

12

Eating on the Run Weight-Loss Guide

"I'm too busy to diet, but I hate my weight."—
medical sales representative

Don't you wish you could dream or melt your fat away? Of course, you know this is impossible. There are no overnight miracles or cures for weight loss (despite what the ads say).

Yet many intelligent people embark on bizarre diets, often because they want the pounds off yesterday. Numerous diet books (some good, others not good) have hit the bestseller list. A Los Angeles talk-show host remarked that diets are second only to sex in popularity among discussions in his office.

WHY DIETS OFTEN FAIL FOR PEOPLE ON THE GO

Quick diets with ultraquick solutions usually just put your lifestyle on hold, temporarily. You don't learn how to deal with potential problems such as eating out, social settings, travel, or sweet tooths; with these diets you are merely postponing these situations.

As a result, you may lose the weight, but not for long. When the diet is over, you revert back to your real lifestyle and easily regain the weight. You have only deferred the problem, and it quickly catches up with you.

Busy people may be more vulnerable to quick weight-loss gimmicks that are not effective in the long term. Combine desperate people with questionable (at best) entrepreneurs, and you have the latest weight-loss fad. You can save time by steering clear of fad diets.

Here are some tips to prevent you from becoming the newest notch on the belt of futile approaches to fat loss:

1. If it sounds too good to be true, it probably is.
2. If it promises fast weight loss, you will probably be losing the wrong kind of weight—water. Two cups of water weighs one pound. To lose 10 pounds of fat in a week, you would have to eat 5,000 less calories per day! (One pound of fat is equal to 3,500 calories.) Crash diets promote water and lean-tissue loss. But the real tragedy is that when you (inevitably) gain the weight back you don't gain back muscle—you gain fat. You become fatter than before even though you are back to your original weight.
3. A complete program should include a combination of lifestyle management, exercise, and balanced food intake.

   Here are some clues to see if your diet program is compatible with your busy lifestyle:

   • Does it allow you to eat out (or give guidance on how)?
   • Does it coexist with your eating style (such as grazing)?
   • Does it consider social occasions?
   • Does it consider fast food, frozen food, or convenience food?
   • Does it match your cooking style? For example, if you are suddenly required to cook extravagant dishes with exotic ingredients and you loathe cooking, you could be in for problems.

WHAT ABOUT CONVENIENCE DIETS OR LIQUID DIETS?

While programs such as Jenny Craig or Nutri/System say they incorporate behavior education and sound nutritional habits, there are some problems with such plans. A major problem is that while you are eating packaged diet food you are not living in the real food world, making decisions about what to eat, and so forth.

For example, some of my business clients have told me how they would pull out their diet cuisine food packets in a restaurant while their clients dined on regular menu fare. Needless to say this behavior did not last long. It was not realistic, and it ignored the core issue—how to order in a restaurant without doing your waistline in.

The programs may discuss these kinds of issues or lecture on behavior change, but all the while you are on some canned or packaged diet. This does not seem effective. It's like trying to learn how to play the guitar by hearing someone describe how to do it—without the benefit of actually playing or struggling to reach a chord with your own fingers.

Liquid diets such as Slim-Fast, which replaces one or two meals, again seem easy but ignore the real eating problems. I fear that if a person is continually having to lose the same 10 pounds over and over again (wedding, post-vacation, class reunion, and so forth), this could set the stage for yo-yo dieting, in which lost weight keeps coming back and it becomes more difficult with each diet to lose weight.

Let me say, however, that some people will attest, ''All it took to lose weight for good was Nutri/System or Slim-Fast.'' I wish them well, but the odds are just not good with these approaches.

If you are trying to save time, scrapping one diet only to have to go on another is a waste of your time and could damage your metabolism.

THE LIFE SPAN OF A DIET

Sadly, study after study has shown that the more you diet, the harder it becomes to lose weight. Your body becomes more resistant to dieting. Consider what these studies have shown:

- High school wrestlers who go on severe diets develop a lower metabolism rate—and these are young healthy males!
- Rats put on a yo-yo diet regain the weight quicker, and it takes them longer to lose the weight.

It seems that the body can tolerate only a certain amount of dietary assaults; then it revolts. When you go on a crash diet, your body thinks you are starving it. It doesn't know that the lack of food is only temporary. As a result, it adapts by going into a starvation mode and conserving every calorie you give it. Meanwhile your metabolic rate slows down, which lowers your calorie requirement and makes it even easier to regain any lost pounds.

What does this mean? An effective weight-loss plan requires a real commitment, so choose carefully.

D-i-e-t is truly a four-letter word. Diets can wreak havoc on your body and waste your valuable time. They fail to teach you eating habits. *Diet* sounds so negative. I do not like to use this term for weight management.

EATING ON THE RUN
WEIGHT-MANAGEMENT STRATEGIES

It's important to begin with a good mind-set. Here are two keys.

Progress Not Perfection.   This positive mind-set will get you through tough times and help you to keep perspective. Remember, minor eating indiscretions will not affect your health or weight—it's what you do routinely. Believing that you must be perfect with your eating habits can often send you into a downward spiral that results in throwing in the towel. Here's an example: "I ate one piece of cake. I blew it. So I might as well have a couple of more slices." Avoid these self-defeating thoughts. Focus on your progress.

No Forbidden Foods.   Surprised? Here's why. If I told you, "Do not think of an elephant, and that elephant (which you are not thinking about) is pink," what would pop into your mind? A pink elephant! Likewise, if I were to dictate, "No ice cream, no cake, no cookies," all you would think about would be these forbidden foods. In fact, one patient told me about her dieting past: Her favorite part of the diet was going off it; she would plan for weeks what she would pig out on.

A theory gaining in popularity presents another argument against declaring certain foods off-limits. The restraint theory says that people who are very rigid and restrained about what foods they eat tend to overeat when a disinhibitor comes along. A disinhibitor can be an event or situation that causes a person to give in to a forbidden food. Giving in may happen for the following reasons:

1. A person may feel the urge to indulge now because the diet begins again on Monday (as usual), and this may be the last opportunity to ever have this food again.
2. The person probably cannot eat a forbidden food without rationalizing or feeling guilty and therefore has never truly enjoyed the food. (Rather he or she will often eat it fast, almost denying they are even eating—as if to hurry up and get on with the guilt.)

3. The person has felt deprived for so long that after one bite of the forbidden food, he or she doesn't know how to handle it and loses control.

The point behind no forbidden foods is learning how to work with your problem. Confront the food issue head on. For example, 5 scoops of ice cream don't taste any better than 1, so why have a heaping bowl? Chances are your taste buds are frozen by the time you are down to the last few scoops. Or you may need to learn to eat only when you are hungry and to stop when you are comfortable (instead of full).

STRATEGIES FOR TAKING ACTION

Let's look at some quick but effective strategies that, if practiced consistently, could help you achieve your ideal weight—without the hassle of being on a diet.

Getting Started

There are four basic steps to help you with your core areas, but first you need to know where your problems are.

Step 1.   Identify your problem area by keeping a food journal (also referred to as self-monitoring). This activity alone can curtail your eating. Be sure to include a weekend. Many of my patients will say, "But I don't eat the same on weekends. It's not typical." Keep in mind that in one year there are 52 weekends, or 104 days, of weekend eating. It does count!
    Note in your journal the following:

- Place where you ate (kitchen, office, bedroom)
- Duration (how long it took you to eat)
- Mood when you ate (bored, stressed, angry)
- Simultaneous activity (watching television, reading)
- Whether you left your plate "clean"

What are your eating trends? Your record may reveal that you "wolf down" all your meals in 10 minutes, even when you are not racing against the clock. Or you may notice that every time you feel under stress, you find your hand in a box of cookies. Perhaps you notice you tend to gorge nonstop once you arrive home from work.

Step 2. Identify your priority areas that you want to change. Then look over the six action that follow and decide which would most affect your eating. (You want to go for the jugular. Begin with the changes that will have the most impact, and then fine-tune the other areas.)

Step 3. Choose only one or two changes per week. For example, ''I will walk four times a week.'' If you try to do everything at once, you may feel frustrated and overwhelmed. Do not move on to another area until you feel your new habits are established.

Step 4. Monitor your progress by tracking your habit changes on the tracking form (see Figure 12.1). I find this to be a very useful tool, and I think you will, too. It allows you to see your progress and spot trends.

Changing What Triggers You to Eat

Different situations (stimuli) can trigger your eating. For some people it might be emotional hunger. For example, stress, boredom, or anger might trigger some people to eat. For others, grocery shopping on an empty stomach might cause impulse buying of goodies that eventually end up . . . you know where. Recognizing your ''food triggers'' can help you cope with your situation and avoid a fat splurge. (This is where a food journal is particularly insightful.)

Action Strategies

Once you have identified your food triggers, it is time to take action. The following are some strategies that might help.

Emotions.

1. Devise a list of activities to cope with your emotions. These activities should be incompatible with food. Keep the list handy and ''on call.'' For example, to combat stress, put these activities on your list: take a bath, get a massage, get a manicure, listen to your favorite music.
2. Always ask yourself, Am I hungry?

Social Pressure and Parties.

1. Mentally practice ways to decline food offers.
2. Eat a small snack before going to a party.
3. Mentally plan how much alcohol you will drink.

Figure 12.1   Tracking my habit changes

+ = Achieved
0 = Not achieved

Goals	Date																																									
Example: Walk 30 min 5 x week	+	0	+	+	0	+	+	0	+	+																																	
1																																											
2																																											
3																																											
4																																											
5																																											
6																																											
7																																											
8																																											
9																																											
10																																											
11																																											
12																																											
13																																											
14																																											
15																																											
16																																											
17																																											
18																																											
19																																											
20																																											

4. Stretch out alcoholic beverages by adding lots of ice; adding a no-calorie mixer such as mineral water; or making your own drink.
5. Carry on conversations away from food.

Grocery Shopping.

1. Carry just enough cash for planned purchases.
2. Shop from a list.
3. Shop when you are *not* hungry.
4. Place groceries out of reach on your journey to prevent the temptation to nibble.
5. Bypass the chips, cookies, and candy aisles.
6. Store food out of sight.

Cooking.

1. Don't nibble while preparing food.
2. Try chewing gum.

Impulse Control.

1. Plan your snacks and keep them handy.
2. Plan your meals.
3. Go no longer than 5 hours without eating.

Serving and Storing Food.

1. Use smaller dishes and glasses.
2. Avoid being the food server.
3. Keep serving dishes off the table (leave them in kitchen).
4. Put leftovers away immediately.
5. Keep food out of sight (not in candy dishes).

Changing the Act of Eating

Changing just one or two ways that you eat can often significantly reduce your intake—without making you feel deprived. You may have heard of some of the following action ideas before, but have you ever actually tried them? Knowledge and action are two different things. Obviously, you must have knowledge first. If you do not act on that knowledge, however, you are no better off.

Unfortunately, life in the "fax lane" often breeds fast eating techniques that can be hard to turn off. Just because your life is fast-paced does not mean that every meal has to be gulped down in no time flat.

On the days when you do have a little extra time to sit and eat a meal, try these strategies and you will find eating more satisfying.

Action Strategies

Some of these strategies may actually lengthen the duration of a meal. Keep in mind that ideally you should take 20 minutes to eat, about the length of time it takes the brain to realize that your stomach is full.

Beginning.   When possible, do not engage in any other activity when you are eating except talking or listening to music. If you don't focus your attention on eating, you may not notice that your meal has passed by (inside you) and you'll feel as if you have not eaten.

In *Breaking Free From Compulsive Eating*, Geneen Roth describes this situation as ''the sense of being somewhere but not really being there, the 'sorry, how's that again?' feeling. . . . The conversation or event took place, but because our attention wasn't present, it didn't take place for us, in us.''

Designate only one spot for eating (such as the dining room or kitchen). This will help to make you a conscious eater.

During.

1. Swallow completely before beginning your next bite of food.
2. Put your utensils down between mouthfuls.
3. Take smaller bites of food.
4. Relax and enjoy your meal!

Termination.

1. Get rid of the clean plate habit.
2. Rate your hunger level from 1 to 10 before you eat (1 being ravenous, 5 being comfortable, and 10, extremely full, stuffed). Stop eating when you feel you are at a 5, rather than waiting until the plate is empty!
3. Put your napkin on your plate when finished.
4. Or put your eating utensils over the plate when finished.
5. Take your plate to the kitchen sink.
6. Leave the table.

Getting Physical

One critical key to successful weight loss and maintenance is routine exercise. I know you are too busy. But think of it this way, the less fat you have to carry around, the quicker and easier you will be able to move. And with your speedy lifestyle, you could probably use the energy boost that exercise gives you. The net result is that you become stronger and more efficient at ordinary living as well as exercising.

I consider the calorie-burning effect of exercise as a two-for-one deal. First, the act of exercise burns calories; second, the calorie burning is amplified. Exercise helps to increase your metabolic rate, so you burn more calories at other times as well. (Check with your physician before beginning any exercise program.)

Action Strategies

1. Begin exercising. Choose a routine aerobic exercise that you enjoy such as walking, jogging, or biking. Build up to a minimum of three workouts a week of 20 to 40 minutes duration.
2. When traveling try any of the following:
   - Pack a jump rope.
   - Bring walking shoes (a great way to tour a city).
   - Use hotels that have gyms or at least a stationary bike.
   - Check local programming for an aerobic show.
3. Fit activity into your work style:
   - During lunch
   - During breaks
   - After work
4. Need support? Try these:
   - Exercise with a buddy
   - Hire a certified personal trainer

Positive Thinking

As Henry Ford once said, ''Believe you can or believe you can't. Either way you will be right.'' Your attitude can greatly affect how you behave and how you feel.

Action Strategies

1. Dwell on your progress, not your shortcomings.
2. View any setbacks as a learning opportunity.
3. Give yourself three positive messages about yourself daily. (If you don't compliment yourself, who will?)
4. Set realistic goals.
5. Remember, progress not perfection.

Zapping the Fat

What floats on water and has twice the calories of any other energy nutrient? Fat.

Calories are easily disguised in the form of hidden fats. You have seen how much fat is in fast food and frozen entrées. Beware of the fat content of your other food choices; it can make a big difference. For example, drinking one cup of regular whole milk is the equivalent of drinking one cup of nonfat milk with two pats of butter!

New research shows that calories from fat are more easily converted to fat in the body than are calories from protein or carbohydrates. (It makes sense: Fat makes fat!) And not only will you benefit calorically by trimming the fat, but you may also prevent many chronic diseases. (I will discuss this aspect in the following chapter.)

I have compiled a list of alternatives to high-fat foods and ingredients, found in Table 12.1. Try substituting the lower fat options in your favorite recipes. It's a nice way to have your cake and eat it too, literally! And you're more likely to succeed if you can continue to eat your favorite foods with just a few alterations. As you try some of these experiments, keep an open mind.

Try serving a leaner version of a food to guests or family members, but don't tell them about it until after they have tasted it. Otherwise, your healthy announcement may prematurely bias their taste buds.

Don't forget, small fat changes do make a big difference. For example, by eliminating one teaspoon of fat every day for a year, you will save yourself from eating about 4-1/2 pounds of fat!

Use the lowfat suggestions in Table 12.1 for snacks or recipe ingredients. You may be pleasantly surprised.

Quick Tip. If you don't have time to experiment, send your recipe to me in care of *Shape* magazine. Space permitting, I may be able to feature it in my Recipe Makeover column. Write to me at:
Shape
21100 Erwin Street
Woodland Hills, CA 91367

Action Strategies

1. Implement at least two lowfat substitutions (see Table 12.1).
2. Remove excess fat:
   - Drain oil from natural-style peanut butter.
   - Skim fat off soups.

Table 12.1   Alternatives to Help Lower Fat

Instead of	Substitute	Calories saved
Dairy		
1 cup whole milk	1 cup nonfat milk	70
1 cup heavy cream	1 cup evaporated skim milk	621
1 cup sour cream	1 cup nonfat plain yogurt, or	289
	1 cup lowfat cottage cheese + 1 tbsp lemon juice	213
1 cup grated cheddar cheese	1 cup lowfat cheddar	120
8 oz cream cheese	4 oz skim ricotta + 4 oz tofu, or	534
	8 oz Neufchatel light cream cheese	200
Fats		
1/2 cup oil	1/2 cup applesauce, or	907
	1/4 cup applesauce + 1/4 cup nonfat milk, or	914
	1/4 cup applesauce + 1/4 cup oil	454
1 stick margarine/butter	1/2 cup applesauce, or	747
	1/2 cup diet margarine	400
2 tbsp oil	2 tbsp wine or broth	240
1/4 cup gravy	1/4 cup au jus or broth	159
1 cup cream soup	1 cup evaporated skim milk + bouillon cube + 1 tbsp flour	149
1 cup walnuts	1/2 cup walnuts	427
Proteins		
2 whole eggs	4 egg whites	94
1 lb regular ground beef	1 lb ground turkey, or	358
	1 lb extra lean ground beef, or	123
	1 lb diced chicken breast	585
6-1/2 oz tuna in oil	6-1/2 oz tuna in water	182
Miscellaneous		
1 cup chocolate chips	1/2 cup chocolate chips, or	456
	2/3 cup chocolate chips, or	310
	3/4 cup chocolate chips	228
1 cup shredded coconut	1/2 cup shredded coconut	233

- Drain fat from browned meat.
- Remove skin from chicken.

3. Use lowfat cooking techniques: Steam, broil, poach, and use nonstick sprays or nonstick pans.
4. Limit fried foods.

5. Choose primarily foods that have no more than 3 grams of fat for every 100 calories.
6. Remember to limit meat to no more than 7 ounces per day.
7. Choose lower fat foods when eating out (see chapters 6-10).
8. Limit fats (margarine, mayonnaise, salad dressing, oil):
   - Use fruit-only jam instead of butter for toast.
   - Use fat-free salad dressings for bread spreads.
   - Try gourmet vinegars for a savory salad dressing.
9. Be a fat sleuth: Look for hidden fat traps.

Other Food Action Strategies for Weight Control

1. Remember to drink at least 8 glasses of water each day. Water is an essential nutrient. It also helps to remove metabolic wastes and keep you full.
2. Don't forget to eat. I have had overly motivated clients who test the food waters to see how low they can go and nearly starve themselves. This can lead to a food binge.
3. Choose fresh fruit instead of juice. With juices, it is easy to guzzle away your calories.
4. Make food changes gradually.
5. Remember the 6-5-4-3-2 Nutrition Countdown.

13

Disease Prevention

"I was so busy, I didn't care about what I ate—until I found out that my cholesterol was off the chart."—

attorney

What you eat can play a big role in preventing many chronic diseases, such as cancer and heart disease. Yet, as you speed full steam ahead into your schedule, you may be eating the very dietary culprits associated with these diseases. Are you too busy for nutrition? Remember, your health is important. If you do not have time to be sick, make sure your food foundation is solid, one that can reduce your chances of disease.

Two landmark scientific reports (years in the making)—the 1988 *Surgeon General's Report on Nutrition* and the 1989 *Diet and Health Report*—both clearly show that nutrition can make a difference in preventing chronic diseases.

Reading the headlines might lead you to believe that you need only worry about cholesterol to steer clear of the heart-attack track. Actually, you need to think of the big picture. For example, the surgeon general concluded that out of the 10 top killer diseases in this country, diet is related to half of them!

Gearing your eating habits to avoid the disease of the year isn't enough. You need sound nutrition. In this chapter I will summarize and simplify the information about nutrition and health (so you don't have to read the long scientific reports that combined total more than

1,400 pages!). Rest assured, however, that by following the basic 6-5-4-3-2 Nutrition Countdown, you will have a big head start toward disease prevention.

STACKING THE CARDS

I like to think of nutrition and disease prevention as stacking the cards of life in your favor. You have no guarantee that you will never get cancer or heart disease, but you can increase the chances that you won't. By reducing several risk factors, you can take positive control of your life, even with life in the fast lane.

Of course, other factors, such as genetics, your environment, or lack of exercise, may predispose you to chronic diseases. In fact, a combination of all these factors (otherwise known as a multifactorial cause) is probably at the root of these diseases.

CONFUSING STUDIES AND HEADLINES

If you ate according to the nutrition headlines, one week you may be strapping on an oat bran bag, and the next, dousing your toast with olive oil. It's as if your diet is the ball in the tennis match of nutrition research with food companies cheering you on.

Despite the consensus from scientific bodies on dietary risk factors, a lot of confusion exists. One reason is that the exact mechanism of cause in many diseases is still being researched. Also, scientists studying the same topic often use different methods and consequently get different results. For example, there still is not a standard method for determining total dietary fiber in food.

Another problem is that association does not prove cause and effect. For example, hair dryer use, aluminum foil use, and the gross national product are all higher in populations with increased breast cancer rates! But there is no reason to believe that these factors cause cancer. The association is purely incidental.

Adding to this confusion is the diet/medical headline of the week, or the *"New England Journal of Medicine* phenomenon.'' With all due respect to this prestigious medical journal, one study published in *NEJM* does not make or break a theory. It's the preponderance of the evidence (the number of well-designed studies with similar conclusions) that counts. The real conflict is that science focuses on the process, whereas the media focuses more on the results. And sometimes the results are not significant if you look at the method or process of the study design.

Even given the difficulties of scientific research, enough data have been confirmed to warrant changes in the typical American or Westernized diet for healthy living. Keep in mind that further detailed research may fine-tune these recommendations. Let's examine them more closely.

BUILDING A SOLID FOOD FOUNDATION

The following nutrition goals are based on information from several governmental and health organizations, including the U.S. Department of Agriculture, the National Academy of Sciences, the National Cancer Institute, and the American Heart Association. (For a concise summary of their recommendations, see Table 13.1, a-c.)

As you read through the food foundation goals, ask yourself which areas you are doing fine in and which spots you need to work on. And then go to it!

More, More, More

First, the good news. Here are the kinds of foods you need to eat more of. By increasing the good stuff, there will be less room for trouble spots in the diet.

Increase Your Fiber Intake.   Most Americans fall very short in their fiber intake. Aim for a level between 20 to 35 grams per day. (The average American eats only 11 grams of dietary fiber daily.)

One very nice attribute of fiber is that you do not absorb its calories! Fiber is the nondigestible component found in plants, that is, fruits, vegetables, legumes (beans), and grains. We lack the enzyme necessary to break down fiber. Therefore, the body is unable to absorb fiber or its calories. This unique characteristic makes fiber extremely beneficial. It adds bulk to the stool, which is most likely the protective factor against colon cancer. According to a popular theory, increasing stool bulk greatly dilutes any carcinogens that are left over from digesting the food you have eaten. Therefore, the carcinogens are less likely to come into contact with the mucosae that line the intestine. As a result, cancer-causing agents find it much more difficult to cause any damage.

Table 13.1a   Dietary Recommendations From Health Organizations

Organization, policy document	Increase fruits & vegetables	Increase complex carbohydrate (% total calories)	Increase fiber	Increase polyun-saturated fat (% total calories)
California Department of Health Services, 1990: *The California Food Guide*	≥ 5 servings	≥ 6 servings	Yes	Yes
DHHS, 1989: *Year 2000 Objectives for the Nation*	≥ 5 servings	≥ 6 servings bread, cereal, legumes	20-30 g	–
National Academy of Sciences, 1989: *Diet and Health Report*	≥ 5 servings, especially green, citrus, yellow	≥ 55%, ≥ 6 servings bread, cereal, legumes	Through veg-etables, fruits, cereals	< 10%
DHHS, 1988: *Surgeon General's Report on Nutrition and Health*	Yes	Yes	Yes	No
American Dietetic Association, 1988: *Lowfat Living*	5-9 servings	≥ 6 servings bread & cereal	–	Yes
American Heart Association, 1988: *Dietary Guidelines for Healthy American Adults*	–	> 50%	–	≤ 10%
JNC 1988: NHLBI: *Non-pharmaecologic Management of Hypertension*	3,000-4,000 mg potassium from fruits & vegetables	–	–	Useful for control of high blood cholesterol
National Cancer Institute, 1987: *Diet, Nutrition and Cancer: A Guide to Food Choices*	More A- & C-rich, citrus, & cruciferous	More whole grains	20-35 g, avoid supplements	No
NCEP, 1990: *Report of the Expert Panel on Population Strategies for Blood Cholesterol* (NIH pub. no. 90-3046)	Yes	50-60%	–	≤ 10%
USDA/DHHS, 1990: *Dietary Guidelines for Americans*	Yes, ≥ 3 servings vegs., ≥ 2 servings fruit	≥ 6 servings grains	Yes	No
NIH, 1984: *Osteoporosis: Consensus Development Conference Statement*	–	–	–	–
American Cancer Society, 1984: *Nutrition and Cancer: Cause and Prevention*	Yes, especially A- and C-rich	Increase whole grains	–	No

DHHS = Department of Health and Human Services; JNC, NHLBI = Joint National Committee, National Heart Lung Blood Institute; NCEP = National Cholesterol Education Program; NIH = National Institutes of Health; USDA = United States Department of Agriculture.

Note. Table 13.1, a-c, is adapted from California Department of Health Services, 1990.

Table 13.1b   Dietary Recommendations From Health Organizations

Organization, policy document	Limit simple sugars	Reduce total fat (% total calories)	Reduce saturated fat (% total calories)	Limit cholesterol (mg)	Limit sodium (mg)
California Department of Health Services, 1990: *The California Food Guide*	Yes	≤ 30%, 6-8 tsp daily	Yes	–	3,300 mg
DHHS, 1989: *Year 2000 Objectives for the Nation*	–	≤ 30%	≤ 10%	–	Purchase foods low in sodium, reduce salt use
National Academy of Sciences, 1989: *Diet and Health Report*	Yes	≤ 30%	< 10%	< 300	≤ 2,400 mg
DHHS, 1988: *Surgeon General's Report on Nutrition and Health*	Yes	Yes	Yes	Yes	Yes
American Dietetic Association, 1988: *Lowfat Living*	Avoid too many sweets	Use 6 tsp or less	Yes	3 yolks a week	–
American Heart Association, 1988: *Dietary Guidelines for Healthy American Adults*	–	≤ 30%	< 10%	< 300 (4 yolks a week, 1989)	1 g/1000 calories, not to exceed 3,000 mg
JNC 1988: NHLBI: *Non-pharmaecologic Management of Hypertension*	–	–	Useful for control of high blood cholesterol	–	1,500-2,500 mg
National Cancer Institute, 1987: *Diet, Nutrition and Cancer: A Guide to Food Choices*	–	≤ 30%	Yes	–	–
NCEP, 1990: *Report of the Expert Panel on Population Strategies for Blood Cholesterol* (NIH pub. no. 90-3046)	–	≤ 30%	< 10%	≤ 300	–
USDA/DHHS, 1990: *Dietary Guidelines for Americans*	Yes	< 30%	< 10%	Yes	Yes
NIH, 1984: *Osteoporosis: Consensus Development Conference Statement*	–	–	–	–	–
American Cancer Society, 1984: *Nutrition and Cancer: Cause and Prevention*	–	~30%	Yes	–	Limit salt-cured and pickled foods

DHHS = Department of Health and Human Services; JNC, NHLBI = Joint National Committee, National Heart Lung Blood Institute; NCEP = National Cholesterol Education Program; NIH = National Institutes of Health; USDA = United States Department of Agriculture.

Table 13.1c   Dietary Recommendations From Health Organizations

Organization, policy document	Calcium (mg)	Moderate alcohol intake	Maintain weight, exercise	Other recommendations
California Department of Health Services, 1990: *The California Food Guide*	2-3 servings lowfat dairy products	≤ 2 drinks; none if pregnant	Yes; exercise 20 min 3x/week	≥3 bean servings per week; ≤7 oz lean meat
DHHS, 1989: *Year 2000 Objectives for the Nation*	3 servings calcium-rich foods	≤ 2 drinks	Yes	Increase breastfeeding
National Academy of Sciences, 1989: *Diet and Health Report*	RDA (800-1,200 mg)	≤ 2 drinks; none if pregnant	Yes	3,500 mg potassium; keep protein below twice RDA; avoid supplements
DHHS, 1988: *Surgeon General's Report on Nutrition and Health*	Females, increase calcium foods	Yes	Yes	Increase iron-rich foods for high-risk groups
American Dietetic Association, 1988: *Lowfat Living*	2-4 servings lowfat, nonfat milk products	Yes	–	5-7 oz lean meat or alternate
American Heart Association, 1988: *Dietary Guidelines for Healthy American Adults*	–	1-2 oz	Yes	Choose a wide variety of foods
JNC 1988: NHLBI: *Non-pharmaecologic Management of Hypertension*	–	≤ 2 drinks	Yes	–
National Cancer Institute, 1987: *Diet, Nutrition and Cancer: A Guide to Food Choices*	–	Limit	Yes	Variety in diet; avoid frying and high temperature cooking
NCEP, 1990: *Report of the Expert Panel on Population Strategies for Blood Cholesterol* (NIH pub. no. 90-3046)	–	–	Yes	Protein calories 10-20%; ≤6 oz lean meat; use lowfat dairy products
USDA/DHHS, 1990: *Dietary Guidelines for Americans*	2-3 servings lowfat, nonfat milk products	Women ≤ 1 drink; men ≤ 2; none if pregnant or trying to conceive	Yes; lose no more than 1 lb/week	Variety of foods; ≤6 oz lean meat or alternative
NIH, 1984: *Osteoporosis: Consensus Development Conference Statement*	1,000 mg pre-, 1,500 mg postmenopause	–	Exercise	Calcium supplements if needed; vitamin D supplements
American Cancer Society, 1984: *Nutrition and Cancer: Cause and Prevention*	–	Yes	Yes	More fruits/vegs.; avoid supplements; cook healthy

DHHS = Department of Health and Human Services; JNC, NHLBI = Joint National Committee, National Heart Lung Blood Institute; NCEP = National Cholesterol Education Program; NIH = National Institutes of Health; USDA = United States Department of Agriculture.

Fiber also has unique physiological properties. The soluble portion of fiber has been shown to help lower cholesterol and control blood sugar in diabetics. The ever-popular oat bran is high in soluble fiber, and so are other foods, such as beans, fruits, and vegetables. The insoluble fibers are associated with increased bulk and increased transit time.

Other benefits of a high-fiber diet include weight control. Fiber gives a feeling of fullness, without a lot of calories. One study published in 1989 in the *American Journal of Clinical Nutrition* demonstrated that subjects who had high-fiber breakfasts ate less at lunch than their low-fiber counterparts.

A high-fiber diet is also thought to protect against diverticulosis, an abnormal out-pouching of the intestines. Imagine squeezing a long balloon like the ones clowns use to mold shapes. When pressure is applied, the balloon bulges out. Similarly, when people eat a low-fiber diet, they have a very low-bulk stool that causes difficulties with elimination. Unfortunately, once these pouches are formed, food particles can get trapped there, resulting in painful inflammation called diverticulitis.

How do you increase your fiber? Your first impulse may be to add bran or bran tablets, but the solution is not that simple. Different fibers do not act in the same way in the body. Therefore, to reap all the benefits of fiber, you need to eat a variety of them. Here is how:

- Don't rely on fiber supplements.
- Eat whole grain products such as whole wheat bread or brown rice. Be sure to choose breads that list *whole* wheat flour as an ingredient. Otherwise you may wind up with a mostly white flour bread. (White flour is wheat flour that has been refined, or ''defibered.'') Aim for at least four whole grain products out of your six (from the Nutrition Countdown).
- The *Diet and Health Report* advises eating at least 5 servings from a combination of fruits and vegetables. Choose whole fruits and vegetables, rather than their juices, to push up fiber levels.
- Beans are one of the naturally richest sources of fiber. Including them consistently three times a week will give your diet a great fiber boost. Compare the difference between a typical bran serving versus cooked beans in the fiber content, as shown in Table 13.2.

Increase Your Cruciferous Vegetables. These vegetables appear to be protective against colorectal, stomach, and respiratory cancers. Cruciferous vegetables come from the mustard family, also known as the cabbage family. They include broccoli, cauliflower, brussels sprouts, all cabbages, turnips, rutabaga, bok choy, and kohlrabi. By the way, cruciferous vegetables are also a good source of fiber.

These vegetables (as well as other plants) contain xenobiotics, food factors that have no nutrient value but must be excreted by the body.

Table 13.2   Fiber Content in Bran vs. Beans

Food	Total fiber (g)	Soluble fiber (g)
1/3 cup oat bran, uncooked	4	2
1/3 cup rice bran	5.5	1
1/3 cup wheat bran	8	1
1 cup black beans	12	5
1 cup kidney beans	14	6
1 cup pinto beans	12	3

Note. Adapted from *Plant Fiber in Foods* (2nd ed.) by J.W. Anderson, 1990, Lexington, KY: HCF Nutrition Research Foundation. Copyright 1990 by J.W. Anderson.

These compounds may help activate the enzymes in the body that help destroy carcinogens. Study after study consistently has shown that populations who eat higher amounts of vegetables (and fruits) have lower rates of cancer.

Choose Foods Rich in Beta-Carotene, Vitamin C, Selenium, and Calcium.   These nutrients appear to be protective for some types of cancer. The protective nature of the first three nutrients may result from their roles as antioxidants that can trap damaging free radicals (free radicals are made up of oxygen but exert the biological equivalent of rusting). These nutrients also play a major role in a healthy immune system, which in turn may protect against the development of cancer. The benefits of these nutrients have been demonstrated primarily from food sources. Since food contains other protective factors, such as xenobiotics, which compound or nutrient is actually doing the protection is not entirely clear.

A special note about calcium: Low intakes of this mineral contribute to the well-known disease osteoporosis (thinning of the bones), which affects about one out of every four women over the age of 65.

Adequate calcium intake appears important for preventing other diseases, too. Preliminary studies suggest calcium may be protective against colon cancer. And low levels of this nutrient may be related to the incidence of high blood pressure.

All vitamins and minerals are important for good health, but the ones I have just mentioned appear to have the strongest link to preventing chronic diseases. If you follow the 6-5-4-3-2 Nutrition Countdown, you should get a good supply of these nutrients. Here are particularly rich food sources of these nutrients:

- *Beta-Carotene:* Dark green and deep yellow vegetables, such as carrots, broccoli, greens, chard, chicory, kale, spinach, squash, pumpkin, and sweet potatoes, and also tomatoes. Deep yellow fruit, such as apricots, peaches, cantaloupe, nectarines, and mangoes.
- *Vitamin C:* Citrus fruits, such as oranges, grapefruit, and tangerines. Other fruits include strawberries, guava, papaya, and cantaloupe. Vegetables include green and red peppers, broccoli, greens, and cabbage.
- *Selenium:* Tuna, oysters, cod, lobster, Brazil nuts, cashews, molasses, chicken, and whole wheat bread.
- *Calcium:* Dairy products such as milk, yogurt, and cheese (choose the nonfat/lowfat version), tofu (made with calcium sulfate), vegetable greens, broccoli, kale, and salmon with the bone.

Increase Your Variety of Foods.   This is a familiar golden rule. Remember, no one food or food group contains every nutrient you need, so it is important to eat a diversity of foods. And let's take the variety tenet one step further: Get in the habit of rotating the types of fruit and vegetables you eat. Also vary the types and brands of cereal.

Increase "Waist Management" to Maintain a Healthy Weight.   Easier said than done, I know. But being overweight causes a lot of problems other than aesthetic ones. Diabetes, joint problems, heart disease, hypertension, some cancers, and higher death rates are related to being overweight. For some pointers on managing your weight, review chapter 12. Remember, although what you eat is a very important part of the weight balancing act, so is exercise. Don't forget about physical activity.

Make Sure You Have Enough Complex Carbohydrates.   Most Americans fall short of getting complex carbohydrates—the ol' grain group that you are well acquainted with by now. Aim for 6 servings of grains per day (as specified in the Nutrition Countdown).

I am reinforcing this point because, I have found, intellectually most people know that getting enough carbohydrates is important for optimal energy. Yet emotionally, when it comes to eating them, they have trouble getting 4 servings of grains in, let alone the recommended 6! Remember, remember, remember: Carbohydrates are not fattening—it's what you put on them (butter on bread, cream cheese on a bagel).

By the way, eating beans three times a week will also contribute to your complex carbohydrate intake.

Less, Less, Less

Eat less of these food components to help ensure optimal health.

Don't Chew the Fat.   Any way you slice it, fat appears to play a major role in cancer and heart disease. Your daily fat intake should be no more than 30% of your calories. This is the equivalent of about 3 grams of fat for every 100 calories you eat. As a guideline, Table 13.3 shows the maximum amount of fat you can eat without exceeding 30 percent of your total calories.

The type of fat you eat affects your blood cholesterol, and high cholesterol is a factor contributing to heart disease. Saturated fats have the most profound effect in raising cholesterol levels. These fats include all animal fats, hydrogenated oils (like shortening), and tropical oils (coconut oil, palm oil, and palm kernel oil). Saturated fat intake should be less than 10% of your calories. Table 13.3 shows you how many grams of saturated fat you could eat without exceeding this 10% level.

When you do use fat, choose oils low in saturated fats because they tend to lower cholesterol. These fats are oils from nontropical plant sources and are liquid at room temperature. They include canola, safflower, corn, sunflower, olive, and soy oils.

Regardless of the source of fat, the bottom line is to reduce it. After all, by cutting down on your total fat intake, you will almost always

Table 13.3   **Maximum Daily Fat Levels**

The maximum fat goals: Total fat should be no more than 30% of calories, and saturated fat intake should be no more than 10% of fat calories. Here's what this means:

Calories	Maximum total fat (g)	Maximum saturated fat (g)
1,000	33	11
1,200	40	13
1,500	50	16
1,800	60	20
2,100	70	23
2,400	80	26
2,700	90	30
3,000	100	33

simultaneously reduce your saturated fats. You might want to look through the suggestions for cutting down on fat given in previous chapters to help you identify the lower fat choices compatible with your eating style.

Limit Cholesterol. High blood cholesterol levels are significantly related to increased rates of heart disease. Several scientific bodies recommend a maximum dietary intake of 300 milligrams of cholesterol per day.

You get cholesterol in two ways. Your body makes cholesterol in the liver, and you get it from the foods that you eat. Only animal products contain cholesterol. Yet with the bombardment of "no cholesterol" claims, it is easy to believe that cholesterol was once in foods like peanut butter and vegetable oils. Plant products never had cholesterol!

Here are some quick tips to make sure your cholesterol remains in check:

1. Make sure your intake of meat (anything with fins, furs, or feathers) does not exceed 7 ounces daily. Preferably, keep it in the lower range of 4 ounces. This is how it can be done, easily:
   - Substitute meat-based meals with bean-based meals.
   - Use meat more as a condiment rather than as the "main event," in dishes like spaghetti.
   - Limit meat to just one meal rather than two meals per day.
2. Limit egg yolks to four or less per week, including those used in cooking. Get in the habit of "poke-a-yolk." Treat eggs like olives and get rid of the yolk. Instead, use two egg whites in place of each whole egg in cooking.
3. Lighten up the cheese. Make it a habit to use only lower fat varieties (less than 5 grams fat per ounce). This will usually mean hold the cheese when eating out.
4. Use nonfat or lowfat dairy products.

Limit Salt, Sodium, and Cured Foods. High-sodium diets have been associated with high blood pressure and cancer of the stomach and esophagus.

The recommended maximum intake is 6 grams of salt (sodium chloride), which is equivalent to 2,400 milligrams of sodium daily. Ideally, 1,800 milligrams of sodium or less would be a healthier goal.

"But I don't use salt," you say. Most of the sodium in U.S. diets does not come from the salt shaker! About 75% of sodium consumed is in the form of processed foods. Only 15% of sodium intake is from using salt at the table or in cooking. Surprised? Consider that foods such as frozen waffles and instant pudding have about 500 milligrams of sodium per serving—and they don't even taste salty.

Cured foods are not only high in sodium; they contain nitrites. Nitrites can be converted to a carcinogen called nitrosamines. This reaction is thought to take place primarily in the stomach, although it still has not been verified in humans. Paradoxically, nitrites are an important compound because they prevent the growth of the potent bacterium *Clostridium botulinum*, which has a deadly toxin that causes botulism.

Eating large quantities of salt-preserved or salt-pickled foods may also increase the risk of stomach cancer. If you focus on keeping sodium within the 2,400 milligram goal, this will limit cured and salt-preserved foods.

The following steps will help you reduce your sodium intake:

- Read food labels carefully, and check for sodium content.
- Decrease your use of salty condiments such as soy sauce, steak sauce, pickles, and olives.
- Use herbs and spices in cooking more often and rely less on added salt. Try dry mustard, garlic powder, onion, lemon, cumin, dill, and other sodium-free seasonings.
- Limit consumption of cured and smoked meats, and instead buy plain or oven-roasted meats.

Limit or Omit Alcohol Intake.   Heavy drinkers are at risk for developing cancer of the mouth, larynx, esophagus, and liver. Beer is strongly associated with rectal cancer. Excessive alcohol drinking also increases the risk for heart disease, high blood pressure, chronic liver disease, nervous disorders, and nutritional deficiencies.

For those who drink, the upper limit should be no more than 2 drinks a day. One drink is equivalent to

1 can of beer;
1 small glass of wine; or
1/2 ounce of hard liquor.

If you are trying to cut calories, alcohol is a good place to start. Of course, pregnant women should abstain from alcoholic beverages.

Limit Caffeine.   The bottom line is caffeine is a drug (you are probably quite aware of its stimulant effect).

The studies linking caffeine (coffee consumption) with health problems are inconsistent. Some show that caffeine is associated with elevated cholesterol, fibrocystic breast disease, rapid heart beat, and some cancers. But it seems for every study showing detriment, there is another showing no relationship! In 1986, the *American Journal of Epidemiology* reported on a 25-year follow-up study of over 3,000 people. Men who drank more than 5 cups of coffee daily showed an increased mortality rate. However, no association was found for women.

Obviously, the scientific jury is still out on caffeine. But in most studies showing an association between caffeine and a health risk, it's at a level of over 4 cups of coffee a day.

Aim for a caffeine level of no more than 200 milligrams per day (about 12 ounces of coffee).

Limit Sweets (Sugar, Honey, and Other Sweeteners). Sugar and sweeteners supply very little in the way of nutrients (an exception is blackstrap molasses) but can add substantial calories. Hence the common description, "empty calories." And many sugary foods, such as cake, ice cream, and doughnuts, are also high in fat.

The average sugar consumption per person is nearly 24 teaspoons per day, about 21% of a typical calorie intake. Too high!

"I don't add sugar to my foods," you say? Consider that a typical soda pop has 9 teaspoons of sugar, one cup of fruit yogurt has about 6 teaspoons of sugar, and one granola bar has about 4 teaspoons of sugar. You can see how this adds up.

Fortunately, sugar is not linked with deadly diseases although eating sweets is certainly related to dental caries. Try these tips to reduce your sugar intake:

- Choose canned fruits packed in their own juice, or with no sugar added.
- Instead of soda, try mineral water, nonfat or lowfat milk, iced tea, or juice.
- Sweet tooth? Make it count. Increase the nutrient density by choosing foods that have some nutritional value, such as frozen yogurt or a bran muffin.
- Reduce your added sugar by 25% (the food will still taste good but will have less sugar).
- Increase use of sweet spices, such as cinnamon, nutmeg, and allspice.

NUTRITION GOALS SUMMARY

Essentially, the Eating on the Run nutrition goals are simply the 6-5-4-3-2 Nutrition Countdown, with emphasis on quality food choices. Choose foods that are low in fat, cholesterol, sodium, and sugar, and high in fiber.

14

Are Vitamins a Quick Fix?

"But I really feel a difference."—
client who takes supplements

Feeling a little draggy? Need extra energy? Will popping some vitamins give you a little perk? Can supplements be an effective nutritional shortcut to optimal health? If you decide to take a supplement, which is best? Read on.

ENERGY BOOSTERS?

When you are on the run, more often than not, "normal" fatigue (not due to illness) is related to the following:

- Inadequate sleep
- Not enough food (or the wrong types)
- Going long periods without eating
- Overtraining (exercise)
- Mental stress

Taking a vitamin pill will not make up for sleep deprivation, stress, or lack of eating. If it were only that easy, I would be the first in line with my hand out and my mouth open.

Vitamins themselves do not supply energy; only calories do. Remember calories come from carbohydrates, protein, and fat. Vitamins do help convert these energy nutrients into the biochemical energy that the body needs.

If fatigue comes from burning the candle at both ends, your best solution is a combination of sleep, stress management, and conscious eating, rather than simply taking a vitamin.

Think of it this way. When endurance athletes want extra energy for performance, they are advised to carbohydrate load, not vitamin load.

NUTRITION SHORTCUT

An unhealthy diet with a vitamin/mineral supplement still remains an unhealthy diet. A supplement is no excuse for poor eating, but it can easily become a crutch if you are not careful.

The core nutritional problem in this country is not one of deficits but rather excesses, the "too syndrome": too much fat, too much cholesterol, and too much sodium. You have already seen that these particular dietary components have the most damaging effect on your health. A supplement will not counteract a diet that is high-fat, high-sodium, high-cholesterol, or low-fiber.

POPULAR MISCONCEPTIONS

The following are some other popular misconceptions people have about vitamin/mineral supplements:

Vitamin supplements are natural. The most natural form in which a vitamin can be found is food! To get the vitamin or mineral into pill form requires many extraction processes and then condensation into a tablet—this is far from natural.

A good supplement will meet all your nutritional needs. No such single supplement exists because everything you need could not fit into a gulp-size pill. In addition, many food factors that enhance nutrient absorption are found only in food. Other nutrients and food factors may not have been discovered or identified yet. Supplement companies can put only the known nutrients into their pills. For example, phytochemicals, naturally occurring compounds in plant foods, have been found to be cancer-fighting. The National Cancer Institute is working on a study to identify these agents. To date, there are over 9,229 species of plants containing these food factors, and they do occur in ordinary foods. Broccoli, for example, has about 34 phytochemicals. But, until they are identified and isolated, phytochemicals cannot be added to supplements.

By relying on supplements, you may be missing out on some key nutrients. According to some new and exciting research it appears that the trace mineral boron is essential to humans. This mineral is most abundant in apples, pears, grapes, and many vegetables, but it is not commonly found in a multivitamin/mineral supplement. So if you decided to skip on the fruits and veggies because you had your supplement, you may have missed out on some boron. To date there is no Recommended Dietary Allowance (RDA) for boron because there is not enough data.

People under stress need more vitamins.   Emotional stress does not significantly increase nutrient needs. However, stressful times can often put food low on the priority list, resulting in poor eating habits and less energy. Hence, a vicious cycle is weaved.

Everyone needs a supplement to prevent nutritional deficiencies.   If you eat a healthy diet (as has been described throughout this book), you do not need vitamin supplements. Unfortunately, powerful advertising techniques can cultivate a nutritional inferiority complex in even the most rational person.

Nutritional supplements are safe.   As toxicologists are fond of saying, it's the dose that makes the poison. Nutrients in high levels can be dangerous. For example, the mineral iron can be fatal in large doses. That's why you see the warning labels on children's vitamins. Iron overdose is one of the most common causes of poisoning in children. Megadosing is discussed in the next section.

MEGADOSING

Some people unknowingly play Russian roulette with their metabolism. Despite the fact that vitamins and minerals sound so natural and healthy, they are not necessarily innocuous. These supplements are among the most commonly abused drugs in this country when taken in megadoses. A megadose is generally considered to be 5 times the RDA of fat-soluble vitamins (A, D, E, K) or 10 times the RDA of water-soluble vitamins (such as B-6).

Megadosing can be hazardous to your health, which is a sad irony because many people think they are improving their health by taking high doses of supplements. More, in this case, is not better.

The body handles high doses of nutrients similarly to drugs. As a result, extra metabolic stress is placed on the liver and kidneys. It may take years for the damage to show up.

Rob-Peter-to-Pay-Paul-Principle

One way supplements can hurt your nutrition is the rob-Peter-to-pay-Paul principle. In this situation, high doses of one nutrient displace another. For example, large doses of zinc inhibit copper absorption. High calcium supplements can impair iron absorption. Large doses of the essential amino acid (EAA) leucine can inhibit the uptake of another EAA, isoleucine. This is why singular supplements, such as single doses of zinc or vitamin B-6, can especially upset your metabolic machinery. They represent a hit-or-miss approach to nutrition that also throws you off balance.

Nutrients must be kept in balance (there's a familiar word), or you may induce a deficiency state. That's unlikely to happen if you are getting your nutrients through nature's best package, food (or, if necessary, through sensible supplementation—I will discuss how to go about this later).

Toxicity

It is widely known that fat-soluble vitamins, especially vitamins A and D, can be toxic in large amounts because they are stored in the body. Even levels of 3 to 5 times the RDA for vitamin A may cause birth defects when taken by the mom during pregnancy.

Some water-soluble vitamins also have been shown to be hazardous in large amounts. For example, vitamin B-6 has been shown to cause symptoms of paralysis and other dysfunctions of the nervous system in women taking large doses.

One of the best examples of toxicity based on dose is the water-soluble vitamin niacin, which also has been legitimately classified as a drug. Niacin is considered a therapeutic drug when given in large doses to help lower cholesterol and triglycerides. But as a drug, niacin also has side effects, documented in clinical trials, such as gout, liver problems, aggravation of peptic ulcers, and elevated blood sugar. Therefore, if niacin is taken to help control cholesterol, it should be done with the supervision of a physician who can monitor for any potential side effects.

Withdrawal Symptoms and Dangers

When discontinuing megadose supplements, it is a good idea to pay careful attention to the process. Stopping abruptly might cause problems. For example, you could induce vitamin C withdrawal symptoms if you suddenly stopped taking it—resulting in symptoms of scurvy (such as bleeding gums).

In most cases, your body begins to compensate for high doses of a vitamin by destroying and excreting (if possible) the vitamin at an increased rate. Therefore, do not throw away your meganutrients. Instead, gradually decrease the dosage. For example, you could begin by taking one pill every other day instead of daily. This tapering process is one that doctors use to wean patients off drugs that are no longer needed.

WHO CAN BENEFIT FROM A SUPPLEMENT?

How can you tell if you need a supplement? Simply evaluate your food intake using the 6-5-4-3-2 Nutrition Countdown. Ask yourself the following questions: Are there any areas in which I chronically fall short? How can I resolve these problem areas? What foods am I willing to eat? If you just need a little consistency in your eating, refer back to the beginning chapters.

You may benefit from a supplement (but not a megadose) if you fall into any of the following categories:

- Devout vegetable hater
- Perpetual dieter, consuming less than 1,500 calories per day
- Pregnant or breastfeeding woman
- Strict vegetarian or not eating an entire food group
- Elderly, with difficulty eating and preparing food

HOW TO CHOOSE A SUPPLEMENT

The majority of people seldom need supplements for optimal nutrition. However, if you fall into one of the above nutritional risk categories or if you're still working on consistent eating, follow the guidelines for safe supplementation.

Choose a supplement that does not exceed 100% of the RDA. The RDA is not a minimum amount on which you barely squeak by. Based on age group and sex, the RDA level for nutrients is padded with a generous safety factor, so nearly everyone who consumes 100% of the RDA gets more than enough of a nutrient.

The 1989 National Academy of Science's *Diet and Health Report* also recommended avoiding supplements exceeding 100% of the RDA, based on studies of the relationship between diet and chronic disease. Keep in mind, a 100% multivitamin/mineral supplement, combined with the food you are eating, will most likely give you a nutrient intake approaching double the RDA.

Choose a multivitamin/mineral supplement rather than a "bullet approach" of single nutrient pills. However, most of these once-daily types have very little room for calcium in their tablets, so women consuming less than 3 servings daily of lowfat dairy foods should consider taking a separate calcium pill.

Beware of designer supplements. These types of supplements generally cost more than others and contain ingredients that sound like nutrients but are actually irrelevant additives with no nutritional value. For example, choline, inositol, and carnitine are compounds made in ample amounts by the body and therefore do not need to be supplied by the diet or supplements.

You may pay more for vitamins described as "natural." This is an unnecessary expense because a vitamin is a vitamin, regardless of its source. Your body cannot tell the difference between a laboratory-made vitamin and one derived from a plant.

Read the label carefully. Some supplements, especially chewable vitamins, may contain hidden sugar and fat. Compare different supplement brands. If they are identical in the amounts of nutrient composition, buy the least expensive.

Do not rely on supplements as a nutritional shortcut. Remember, pills do not contain nature's special balance of nutrients and "food factors" found in food, nor do they make up for poor eating habits.

15

Kids on the Run

"More than two thirds of children under the age of 13 prepare one or more meals per week without supervision."—
American Frozen Food Institute survey

If Mom and Dad are on the run, who's feeding the kids? Let's not forget that children have busy schedules, too—be it dance lessons, soccer practice, or baseball—which means that the whole family is often on the run.

The kids may be coming home to an empty house and preparing their own snacks or meals. Even when parents are home, children may be subject to the same challenges as adults face, such as fast foods and frozen meals. Kids also face food hurdles created by the food industry specially for children.

KID GIMMICKS

Kid gimmicks abound, from edible cartoon characters to toys buried in the food. Challenges to kids go beyond ordinary label reading—it can be a matter of out-and-out bribery.

For years the kid-food wars were primarily the domain of the cereal aisles. But the specialty kid market has grown. Now several kinds of food are targeted at kids:

- Flintstones vitamins
- Ghostbusters cereal
- Looney Tunes frozen meal
- McDonald's Happy Meal (with prize)
- Pac Man canned meal
- Teenage Mutant Ninja Turtles ''fruit'' drinks

Get the picture? The trend is for best-selling toys, cartoons, or movies to become food, of sorts. Too often this leads to a lot of razzle, without the important nutritional dazzle.

That's unfortunate because the growing years are a critical time for getting good nutrition. And statistics show some rather shocking facts about our children's health. For instance, in the United States childhood obesity doubled over the past decade. And between 20% and 40% of school-age children have high cholesterol levels. The American Academy of Pediatrics reported that nearly 40% of 662 school-age children screened in Westminster, California, had elevated cholesterol levels. Results of an ongoing Dietary Intervention in School-Age Children (DISC) study revealed that 40% of 5,000 school-age children in Chicago had elevated blood cholesterol levels.

These examples show that we should not take our children's health for granted. We'll look at the best strategies for feeding kids on the run and the best picks among kiddie foods. But first, a few words on building a good nutrition foundation.

NUTRITION FOUNDATION

The eating principles for children are similar to those for adults. Here's a quick summary:

1. Food Groups: The Nutrition Countdown system still applies (for detailed breakdown by age see Table 15.1).
2. Snacks are important (more details to come).
3. For kids under age 2, fat should not be restricted.
4. Gentle reminder: The growth curve (height and weight) should always be monitored. Sudden plateaus or shifts can be a red flag. If a child does not get adequate calories, his or her growth could be stunted. Do not hesitate to consult your pediatrician or a registered dietitian who specializes in child nutrition.

Table 15.1   Nutrition Countdown for Kids

Recommended number of servings each day

			Protein			
Age group (yrs)	Grains	Fruits/ vegetables	Lean meats (oz)	Beans	Lowfat dairy	Fats (tsp)
Toddler [a]						
1-2	7-11	5-9	3-4	3/wk	2	2
2-3	7-11	5-9	3-4	3/wk	2	6
Children						
4-6	7-11	5-9	3-4	3/wk	2	8
7-10	7-11	5-9	5-7	3/wk	2	8
Young Adult						
Female						
11-18	7-11	5-9	5-7	3/wk	3	8
Male						
11-14	7-11	7-9	7	3/wk	3	8
15-18	9-11	7-9	7	3/wk	3	10

Note. From California Department of Health Services, 1990.

[a]Provide half-size servings. For children under age 2 provide whole milk only.

TAMING THE SNACK ATTACK MONSTER

Snacking is vital to growing children to ensure they get enough calories to support their growing needs. It's hard for kids to get all their nutritional needs in three meals because of their small stomachs and appetites. Choosing the right snacks is key. Here are some tips for the tiny snack rampages.

Keep It Fun.   Most kids could care less about nutrition. Taste and fun are their most important considerations (which is apparent when you watch food commercials targeted at children).

Have Snacks Available.   Kids are natural grazers, so they tend to eat what is handy. If the cupboards are bare, the kids are more likely to hit the local candy outlets.

Get the Kids Involved. This will usually save time. Give the child choices. For example, let the child choose what kinds of fruits he or she would like to snack on. See Table 15.2 for snacking ideas.

Table 15.2   Snack Alternatives for Kids

Here's a list of snacking ideas that are pleasing to tiny palates and are great nutrition boosters.

Instead of	Try
Candy	Peanut butter (old-fashioned type with no added sugar, drain the oil) on bananas or celery, peanut butter sandwich with fruit-only spread, dried fruit.
Chips, crackers	Baked corn tortilla chips, popcorn rice cakes, raw vegetables, lowfat crackers, unbuttered popcorn.
Cookies	Whole wheat apricot bars, vanilla wafers, gingersnaps, graham crackers, oatmeal.
Cream-filled snack cakes	Specialty flavored breads, such as banana nut, pumpkin, zucchini, poppy seed, apricot, or raisin. Try Hula Bagel (one-minute meal, chapter 19).
Dip	Mix half yogurt and half blenderized cottage cheese. Then add favorite dip mix. Serve with raw vegetables or lowfat crackers.
Doughnuts	Variety bagels, such as raisin, apple, cinnamon, blueberry, or strawberry.
Gelatin	Prepare with juice instead of water and add fruit slices.
Ice-cream sundae	Nonfat frozen yogurt or lowfat ice cream, topped with crushed fresh fruit such as berries; juice bars; ice-milk bars.
Pie	Baked fruit (i.e., apple or pear); pudding made with nonfat or lowfat milk and sprinkled with crushed graham crackers; applesauce with crumbled graham crackers.
Soda pop	Fruit fizzies. Mix 3 parts juice to 1 part mineral water. Grape, orange, cherry juices work well. (Make sure you are using 100% fruit juice.)

Table 15.3   Sweet Surprises

Food	Added sugar (tsp)
Sweetened fruit drinks (12 oz)	12
Tang (12 oz)	10
Fruit punch (8 oz)	6
Lemonade (8 oz)	6
Gelatin (1 cup)	5
Granola bar (1)	4
Popsicle (1)	4
Fruit rolls (1 roll)	3

Adapted from California Department of Health Services, 1990.

Beware of the Less-Than-Nutritious Surprises.   Juice drinks, fruit bites, and granola bars may grab a child's attention with fun pictures. Don't let the healthy-sounding names deceive you. The level of sugar lurking in some of these treats is quite high. Look at the sugar content of the sweet surprises in Table 15.3.

Sugary snacks can contribute to dental caries (cavities). Even nutritious dried fruit, or any sticky carbohydrate, can promote tooth decay. So it is a good practice to have kids brush their teeth, especially after a sweet or sticky snack.

Another sugary surprise awaits you in the breakfast cereals. For example, one cup of Apple Jacks cereal has about 4 teaspoons of sugar and one serving of Froot Loops has about 3-1/2 teaspoons of sugar. Your best bet here is to read the label on the side panel of the cereal box. Generally, a cereal with 4 grams of sugar or less per serving is considered acceptable (4 grams is equivalent to 1 teaspoon of sugar).

KIDDIE FROZEN CUISINE

Speedy Gonzalez Enchiladas, Daffy Duck Spaghetti—the names may be cute, but frozen meals specially formulated for kids have adult problems: They're high in fat and sodium.

For example, Tyson's Yosemite Sam barbecue chicken has 39% fat calories, Chicken Nuggets from Kid Cuisine by Banquet has 43% fat calories, and My Turkey Meatballs by My Own Meals has 38% fat calories. Here are the ranges of calories, fat, and sodium for these children's food lines (adapted by permission from *Tufts University Diet and Nutrition Letter*, June 1990):

Brand	Calories	Fat (g)	% Fat calories	Sodium (mg)
Banquet Kid Cuisine	240-430	2-23	7-48	390-1000
My Own Meals	210-260	4-11	16-39	440-600
Tyson Looney Tunes Meals	270-390	8-17	26-39	510-740

The Kid Cuisine meals all come with a dessert, usually something chocolate such as a brownie or cookie. With the staggering prevalence of childhood obesity, desserts should not be an obligatory part of a meal. It could condition the child to expect dessert with a meal, an expectation that could continue into adulthood.

Sure, dessert ranks high in kid appeal, but it should be up to the parents to serve it. When dessert comes with the package, it does not give the parent much choice. What parent would say, "Johnny, don't eat that brownie"—as it's nestled in its own little compartment with the rest of the meal.

The better bets for frozen meals are listed in Table 15.4, but they still have rather high sodium levels. Most pediatric dietitians recommend no more than 2,000 milligrams of sodium per day for children (recall the adult maximum is at 2,400 milligrams). I would use these frozen meals as a backup rather than as a staple menu item. You would do well to limit these to no more than once a week. To round out the meal nutritionally add at least the following: nonfat or lowfat milk and raw vegetables such as carrot sticks.

Table 15.4   Better Bets In Kiddie Frozen Cuisine

Frozen food	Calories	Fat (g)	% Fat calories	Sodium (mg)
Banquet Kid Cuisine:				
Cheese Pizza	240	4	15	390
Mini-Cheese Ravioli	250	2	7	730
My Own Meals:				
Chicken, Please	220	4	16	550
My Favorite Pasta	230	8	31	480
My Kind of Chicken	220	7	29	590

(Cont.)

Table 15.4   (Continued)

Frozen food	Calories	Fat (g)	% Fat calories	Sodium (mg)
Snoopy's Choice:				
Chunky Beef Stew	140	2	13	300
Chicken and Pasta with Cream Sauce	230	3	12	500
Chunky Chicken Stew	130	2	14	380
Lasagna with Meat Sauce	280	7	23	490
Macaroni and Beef in Sauce	250	5	18	280
Macaroni and Cheese with Turkey Franks	280	5	16	360
Mini Beef Ravioli in Tomato Sauce	300	7	21	530
Spaghetti with Meatballs and Sauce	270	5	17	370
Tyson Looney Tunes Meals:				
Daffy Duck Spaghetti with Meatballs	320	10	28	650
Tweety Macaroni and Cheese	280	8	26	660
Wile E. Coyote Hamburger Pizza	320	11	31	660
Elmer Fudd Turkey and Dressing	240	7	26	610

Note. Adapted in part by permission from *Tufts University Diet & Nutrition Letter,* June 1990.

Table 15.5   Kiddie Canned Cuisine: Calories, Fat, and Sodium

Canned food	Calories	Fat (g)	% Fat calories	Sodium (mg)
Pac Man:				
Tomato Sauce	150	1	6	830
Meatballs	230	9	35	880
Chicken Sauce	170	7	37	905
Dinosaurs:				
With Mini Meatballs	230	8	31	960
With Cheese Flavor	160	1	6	790
Smurf:				
Beef Ravioli	230	5	20	1,160
Cheese Flavor	150	1	6	830
With Meatballs	240	9	34	900
Tic Tac Toes:				
With Cheese Flavor	160	1	6	870
With Mini Meatballs	240	9	34	1,000

KIDDIE CANNED CUISINE

With names like Pac Man or Smurf, what child could resist these little pasta goodies? While the fat content is not horrific (6-37% fat calories), the sodium content is more than excessive with ranges of 790 to 1,160 milligrams (which is considered high even for adults).

The best bet here is to limit these sodium-loaded meals to rare occasions. If you have to make a choice between canned or frozen pastas, choose frozen. They tend to be lower in sodium (although still not low enough). See Table 15.5 for detailed nutritional information, and you'll see why these foods should be on the ultralimited list.

FAST FOOD: KIDDIE MEAL PACKS

According to a 1990 National Restaurant Association survey, restaurant visits by children under age 6 rose 36% between 1982 and 1988. And fast-food restaurants certainly do their part to clamor for the kid's attention.

Probably no other food industry packs as much fun and hype into eating as fast food. Toys, fun packages, games on the box—some chains even have playgrounds for the little ones. Ever wonder why? The tiniest consumer has a lot of buying power because the parents usually will eat where the children eat.

Let's take a look at what the fast-food chains are packing in for kids. Generally there is a choice of entrées, such as hamburger, cheeseburger, or chicken nuggets. Most meals come with fries and a small drink. Here's a typical example using McDonald's Happy Meal, which includes fries, soft drink, and kid entrée:

Meal	Calories	Fat (g)	% Fat calories
Happy Meal with chicken nuggets	650	28	39
Happy Meal with cheeseburger	670	26	35
Happy Meal with hamburger	620	22	31

See List 15.1 for a description of other kid meals.

One problem with these package meals is the automatic inclusion of fries and soft drink. This could easily condition a child to want fries every time he or she orders in a fast-food place, even without the special kid package. If the kids are fond of fries, there's no harm in occasional fries. But don't let it become a routine order.

List 15.1
Fast-Food Kiddie Packs

Listed below are the kiddie-pack meal options. The entrée with the star is the better choice.

Arby's Adventure Meal
Junior Roast Beef
French fries
Small beverage (okay to substitute milk)

Carl's Jr. Happy Star Meal
*Hamburger, Cheeseburger, or 2 Crisp Burritos
French fries
Small drink (milk or juice okay)

Burger King Kids Club
*Hamburger, Cheeseburger, 6 Chicken Tenders, or 6 Fish Tenders
French fries
Small beverage (soda, shake, milk, or juice)

Long John Silver's
*1 Fish, or 2 Planks, or 1 Fish and 1 Plank
Fryes
1 Hushpuppy
Beverage (okay to substitute milk)

Hardee's
*Hamburger, Cheeseburger, or Chicken Sticks
French fries
Small drink (okay to substitute with milk or juice)
(A spokesperson for Hardee's said that if a parent wishes to purchase the toy separately with a different menu purchase, they will usually accommodate the parent's wishes.)

Kentucky Fried Chicken: Colonel's Kids Meal
*Drumstick or 6 Nuggets
French fries
Soft drink (usually okay to substitute milk but can vary with individual locations)

McDonald's Happy Meal
*Hamburger, Cheeseburger, or 6 Chicken Nuggets
French fries
Small beverage (okay to substitute milk or juice)

Taco Bell Fiesta Meal
*Bean Burrito, Taco, or Soft Taco
Cinnamon Twists/Crispas
Small beverage (okay to substitute milk)

Making the Best of the Fun Meal Packages

As a parent or care giver, you could be in a tug of war with a kid pleading for the Happy Meal. Here are some strategies (I have used them on my own 4-year-old):

1. Don't automatically order the kid special every time you visit, or the child will learn to expect it. Randomize your purchases. Until the kid specials change, I recommend ordering them only on rare occasions.

2. If you buy a kid special, always request milk or juice for the beverage. Most restaurants will accommodate you. Of the typical entrée choices (hamburger, cheeseburger, or chicken nuggets), the small hamburger is the best choice (believe it or not). It is the lowest in fat.

3. Best Bet overall: Order your way. The best bet entrées (from chapter 7) are also the better choices for the kids. The struggle, however, is that there are no toys or games. This can be especially tough when the promotion toy (the premium) is only available through fast-food outlets, so you can't purchase the toy in a store.

4. Be a good model. What you do (in this case eat) speaks much more powerfully than what you tell your kid to do.

CHILDREN'S VITAMINS

Big Bird, Flintstones, Bugs Bunny—sounds like a Saturday morning lineup for television. But these guys are typical brand names in the competitive chewable vitamin wars. Children are one of the largest consumers of vitamins.

Should you be giving your child a daily vitamin? Generally, it is not necessary. Remember, it is possible to get all the essential nutrients from food. But getting kids (especially picky eaters) to eat the right foods can be a challenge. If your child is going through a phase and refuses to eat all vegetables, for example, then taking a general multivitamin may be warranted. Realize, however, that a child's appetite regulation is amazingly keen. As long as your child's growth is within the normal range, he or she is eating enough.

Here are some guidelines:

• Remember that, as with adults, excesses (of fat, cholesterol, and sodium) are the main problem in children's diets, not deficiencies. Therefore, arming Johnny with a vitamin and unlimited fast-food meals does not provide him with optimal nutrition.

- Choose a supplement that does not exceed 100% RDA, and stick with a multivitamin/mineral pill rather than a potpourri of single-nutrient pills.
- Store vitamins out of reach—they can be toxic. (This is an irony because they do taste good.)
- Remember, supplements are not a shortcut to, nor do they teach the foundation of, lifelong healthy eating habits.

SAVORING TIME TOGETHER

In the past, the evening meal was an opportunity for families to enjoy time together. In our busy lives today, we need to remember that making time for the family is important.

Some families have found that the best time to eat together is in the morning. Find what works for you. Consider making a lunch or dinner date with your child; then enjoy a special meal together with no distractions.

We need to be careful not to impose our hurried-eating attitude on the children. Do allow plenty of time for the kids to eat (regardless of age). It might mean getting up an extra 15 minutes earlier because Jenny likes to savor her cereal. Although I see no problem with an adult eating and walking (during tight schedules), this can be dangerous for a child because of the risk of choking.

Perhaps we should take a cue from the Japanese. In their *Dietary Guidelines for Health Promotion*, not only did they advise on what to eat, but they recommended, ''Make all activities pertaining to food and eating pleasurable ones.'' They believe that mealtime should be used as an occasion for family communication. The social aspects of eating are considered as important as the health promotion aspects in Japan.

16

Nutrition for Busy Athletes

"I teach four to five aerobics classes a day and don't have time to eat lunch."—

aerobics instructor

Fitness enthusiasts and athletes seem to have the most difficulty finding time to eat. More often than not, they juggle athletics, work, school, and sleep, while trying to consume enough calories to fuel their bodies for sports activities. When they do find a minute to eat, they don't always choose the best foods.

When I was competing on the track and cross-country teams in college, I would wind up in the team doctor's office every year to "rule out mononucleosis." I was chronically tired, but no medical condition could explain my fatigue. Looking back at my lifestyle, I have no doubt that my problem stemmed from eating too little and inadequate sleep. I would eat only a minimal breakfast because I needed the time for my extra morning run. Then, I normally skipped lunch because it interfered with my afternoon training. By the end of the day, I was literally running on empty. (I was a physical education major back then and not yet nutritionally enlightened.)

Many of the athletes I have counseled—both amateur and professional—have similar difficulties squeezing in time to eat. Serious rec-
reational athletes have time constraints because often they are
training while holding a full-time job.

If your sport or fitness activity takes you on the road, you have the
additional challenge of choosing foods for optimal performance from
a restaurant or fast-food place.

Athletes may need up to several thousand calories a day. To meet
these energy needs, athletes not only must eat but must choose the
right kinds of foods. Otherwise, their performance is likely to suffer.

FOOD FOUNDATION: CARBOHYDRATES

The 6-5-4-3-2 Nutrition Countdown system will serve as a good base-
line food foundation. But if you are involved in training for an hour
or more per day, you will need a more powerful foundation. The
foundation of exercise energy is carbohydrates. To get an idea of your
exercise dependence on carbohydrates, see Table 16.1.

You'll need at least 8 servings of grains and 8 servings of fruits and
vegetables to help fulfill your increased carbohydrate needs.

Table 16.1   Estimated Energy and Carbohydrate Expenditure

	Estimated calories		
Activities	Calories/min	Total calories	CHO (g)
Running			
2 mile	20.0	215	50-55
10 km	17.5	700	150-170
Marathon	15.0	2,800	500-550
Swimming (front crawl)			
200 m	25.0	50	12-15
1500 m	20.0	400	90-100
Cycling			
1 h	17.0	1,020	230-250

Data based on a 70 kg individual (approximately 150 lb). CHO = carbohydrate.

Note. From "Carbohydrates for Exercise: Dietary Demands for Optimal Performance" by D.L. Costill, 1988, *International Journal of Sports Medicine, 9,* p. 5.
Reprinted by permission of Georg Thieme Verlag.

Although variety is important, you do not necessarily need to eat eight different fruits or grains as long as you consume sufficient quantity. For example, one cup of cereal equals 2 grain servings. Most athletes could easily eat four pancakes, which is equivalent to 4 servings from the grain group.

The extra servings from these two groups provide additional carbohydrates, which in turn supply the best types of fuel for exercise. Carbohydrates are stored in the body in the form of glycogen. When you exercise, your body breaks glycogen down to glucose, which fuels the exercising muscles. Numerous studies have shown that when glycogen stores are depleted, exhaustion sets in. An average of 90 minutes of continuous aerobic exercise will usually drain these stores. This critical point of depletion is also known as ''hitting the wall.''

Glycogen stores need to be replenished on a daily basis. If you are training every day and don't eat enough carbohydrates, you may feel chronically fatigued as a result of emptied glycogen. Not only will you feel physically tired, you may suffer psychologically as well. You may begin to doubt your abilities. Or worse, you may think you need to train longer, which would deplete your glycogen stores even further and make you even more exhausted.

You can see that the training diet is very important. Your food foundation will support your training and ultimately your performance. Ironically, many athletes neglect diet until a competition is upon them. You can't suddenly begin working out one week prior to the main event. Similarly, diet needs to be consistent through the long haul—not just right before competition. For some individuals, a training diet will consist of carbohydrate loading every day (I'll discuss this later).

Carbohydrates should be at least 60-70% of your calories. Some experts suggest that if you are involved in prolonged training, you should aim for a carbohydrate level of 400 to 600 grams per day. That doesn't leave a lot of room for fat. A high-carbohydrate diet, then, is also one that is low in fat. Let's look at practical ways to keep those carbohydrates high.

ROAD WARRIORS

Traveling can be a challenge—whether for the college athlete who gets ''meal money'' for the first time, or for the experienced competitor at an out-of-town triathlon.

In previous chapters, I discussed the challenges of eating on the road, particularly the high fat content of readily available foods. But fat-savvy athletes face another special problem: getting enough "carbs." Ironically, in your quest for the lowfat-food grail, you may end up low in calories (energy) and low in carbs (high-octane fuel). For example, a McDonald's Chunky Chicken Salad is low in fat but is also devoid of carbohydrates (and no, fries are not a good source of carbohydrates because of their high fat content).

Here are some guidelines for traveling:

- Order lowfat foods (described in detail previously).
- Order extra carbs (such as rolls, potatoes, cereal, rice, muffins, and juice).
- Stash aside extra carbs. There may be times when you're stuck at an airport or when a meet, match, or game goes on longer than planned and you are caught without food.

Table 16.2 lists some specific best bets for the traveling athlete. This is just a representative guide; there are many other combinations and ways to order "heavy on the carbs."

Table 16.2 Ordering Fast Foods Heavy on the Carbohydrates

These meals range from about 600 to 1,000 calories but can easily be adjusted to meet your caloric needs. All provide at least 60% carbohydrate (CHO) calories.

Food	Calories	CHO (g)
Burger King:		
2 Bagels	554	88
Chunky Chicken Salad	142	8
1 Orange Juice	82	20
Total	**778**	**116 (60% CHO)**
Carl's Jr.:		
BBQ Chicken Sandwich	320	40
10 oz Lowfat Milk	175	16
1 Small Orange Juice	94	21
Lite Potato	250	54
Total	**839**	**131 (62% CHO)**
Hardee's:		
Chocolate Shake	460	85
Grilled Chicken Sandwich	310	34
Total	**770**	**119 (62% CHO)**
Jack-in-the-Box:		
Chicken Fajita Pita	292	29
2 Orange Juices	160	40

Food	Calories	CHO (g)
Side Salad with		
2 pkgs Breadsticks	140	24
1/2 pkt Reduced-Calorie French Dressing	88	13
Total	**680**	**106 (62% CHO)**
McDonald's:		
2 Apple Bran Mufffins	380	92
Chunky Chicken Salad with	140	5
1/2 pkt Lite Vinaigrette Dressing	30	1
8 oz Lowfat Milk	120	12
Total	**670**	**110 (66% CHO)**
Taco Bell:		
2 Bean Burritos (red)	**713**	**109 (61% CHO)**
Wendy's:		
Super Bar		
8 oz Fettuccine Noodles with	760	108
6 oz Spaghetti Sauce	90	21
2 Slices Garlic Toast	140	18
6 oz Orange Juice	80	19
Total	**1,070**	**166 (62% CHO)**
Subway:		
12-in. Turkey Breast on Honey Wheat Roll		
(hold the oil, olives, and cheese)	532	87
8 oz Lowfat Milk	120	12
Total	**652**	**99 (61% CHO)**

PRECOMPETITION OR PREWORKOUT MEAL

What, how much, and when should you eat prior to competition? What about on a day-to-day basis for routine workouts?

Timing

When you eat your meals and snacks can significantly affect your performance both in competition and in routine training. You do not want your stomach to be full of food, which could cause you to feel uncomfortable or nauseated (or even to vomit). This can occur partly because your exercising muscles are competing with your stomach for the blood supply. The more intensely you exercise (sprinting versus slow jogging), the more intensely your muscles need the blood.

At rest, normal blood flow to the digestive tracts is about 25%. During hard exercise, however, only 4% of the blood flow is delivered to the gastrointestinal (GI) system, and 85% is supplied to the muscle. Large meals increase blood flow to the GI tract, diverting it from exercising muscle.

Typically, food empties from the stomach in about 3 to 4 hours after a meal. So ideally you should eat about 3 to 4 hours before working out or competing. Of course, the size and composition of the meal will make a difference on timing.

Composition

You already know that carbohydrates are the best source of energy; they also digest the quickest. High-carbohydrate meals help to "top off" the glycogen stores.

Foods containing protein take a little longer to be broken down. Fat packs a double digestive whammy: It takes the longest to digest, and the presence of fat in the stomach slows down the entire rate of digestion (even for other foods). Bottom line: Aim for high-carbohydrate, lowfat foods.

Quantity

Generally aim for about 500 to 600 calories (with 75 to 100 grams of carbohydrates)—enough to avert hunger and provide energy, yet not enough to put you into gastric distress. Here's an example of a high-carbohydrate meal:

1 cup nonfat milk

1 turkey sandwich (2 ounces turkey, 2 slices bread)

1 cup applesauce

2 graham crackers (rectangles)

This pregame meal has 92 grams of carbohydrates, 515 calories, 60% carbohydrate calories, and only 8% fat calories.

Exceptions

There will be occasions when you don't have the luxury of eating 3 to 4 hours prior to working out. It is still okay to eat, but you will need to decrease the quantity of food proportionately (remember, the goal is to have an empty stomach). For example, 2 hours prior to workout, your meal would be more like a snack, such as one cup of lowfat fruit yogurt, which provides 231 calories, 43 grams of carbohydrates, and only 9% fat calories.

Individual Differences

Being nervous about an upcoming event can explain in part why some seem to have a cast-iron stomach that will tolerate any food and others have to take delicate care as to what goes into their bodies prior to competition.

If you are nervous (such as if you're running a 10K for the first time or if winning has big consequences), blood flow to the GI system decreases. This results in a decreased rate of absorption of nutrients. Motility of the lower GI tract may increase, which can cause diarrhea.

Nothing is worse than having to run into the bathroom instead of across the finish line. This frustrating situation of having put in hours of training only to have it wasted has happened to some of the best athletes.

It was such a chronic problem for me in high school that I had the full upper and lower GI series of tests to rule out a pathological process. What was the finding? "You are normal; it's probably nerves." However, I experienced episodes of diarrhea even during routine training when I was not nervous.

Safe Foods. Safe foods are familiar foods that will agree with you despite your anxiety level. The only way to know which foods are safe for you is to keep a record (remember, eating amnesia is rampant). Through trial and error, using the following method, I was able to eliminate "suspect" foods and put an end to my bathroom blues.

1. Write down what you eat during training and precompetition days.
2. Note how your training or competition went—any gastric distress, nausea, diarrhea?
3. Place a check mark by suspect foods on days that you have GI problems.
4. Circle the foods that consistently agree with you.
5. Generate two column heads: safe and suspect.
   - Place any food with two or more checks in the suspect list. You want to avoid these foods on competition days.
   - Place any food that has been circled two or more times in the safe column. These are foods that should be a safer choice, causing you the least trouble.

If you have a very sensitive GI system, you may want to stay away from high-fiber foods the night before and the day of competition. High-fiber foods increase GI motility, which could exacerbate diarrhea problems. Eating a minimal-fiber precompetition meal could help ensure that little remains in the colon after digestion. Some athletes prefer to opt for liquid meals to guard against GI distress.

I have compiled List 16.1, which shows foods that tend to aggravate a queasy GI. However, I want to emphasize that food tolerances are highly individual. Therefore, do not think of this list as blackballed foods.

List 16.1
Potentially GI-Distressing Foods

Beans	Onions
Boysenberries	Peanut butter
Cabbage	Peanuts
Chocolate	Potato chips
Coffee	Raspberries
Corn	Rich desserts
French fries	Sesame seeds
Ice cream	Strawberries
Olives	Sunflower seeds

No Precompetition Experimenting.   The night before a major competition is not a good time to try new foods or a new diet. You do not know if you will tolerate the food, and the last thing you need is to spend the entire night worrying about indigestion.

Precompetition Meal Checklist

____ Eat safe, familiar foods.

____ Choose high-carbohydrate, lowfat foods.

____ Consider individual food tolerances.

____ Eat meals at least 3 hours prior to training/competing.

____ Scale down your meal to snack size if eating 1 to 2 hours prior to competition.

CARBOHYDRATE LOADING

Carbohydrate loading is a training diet regimen that has enjoyed social and traditional popularity among endurance athletes. It is beneficial for participants in aerobic events lasting more than 90 minutes, such as triathlons, marathons, cycling, and soccer.

Athletes who train 90 minutes or more daily will also benefit from a carbohydrate-loading diet daily. Studies have shown that even elite athletes have difficulty fueling long training bouts on a typical mixed diet of about 50% carbohydrate calories. Keeping day-to-day glycogen levels full also is important to support demands of long training.

Although the term *loading* may imply party time and fun, the goal is to supersaturate glycogen stores with carbohydrates. This delays the onset of fatigue caused by drained glycogen stores.

Carbohydrate-loading protocols have evolved. The latest method of carbohydrate loading, sometimes referred to as the depletion taper protocol, begins by gradually tapering training 6 days before competition, from 90 minutes to no activity (rest). This step is combined with 3 days of a mixed diet (regular training diet) followed by 3 days of high-carbohydrate diet (70% carbohydrate calories). See Table 16.3.

Pitfalls

Despite its popularity and known efficacy, carbohydrate loading may have some inherent pitfalls. Some athletes interpret loading as a license to overeat or to eat whatever foods they want. The goal is to store glycogen, not fat, and overeating any food could easily promote fat storage. I have seen athletes indulge in less-than-optimal food choices, such as ice cream—a high-fat food. The nutritional goal is to

Table 16.3 Depletion Taper Carbohydrate-Loading Protocol

Day	Training	Diet
6	90 minutes	50% CHO
5	40 minutes	50% CHO
4	40 minutes	50% CHO
3	20 minutes	70% CHO
2	20 minutes	70% CHO
1	Rest	70% CHO
0	Competition	

CHO = carbohydrate.

Note. From "Carbohydrates, Muscle Glycogen, and Muscle Glycogen Supercompensation" by W. Sherman, 1983. In *Ergogenic Aids in Sport* (p. 13) by M.H. Williams (ed.), Champaign, IL: Human Kinetics. Copyright 1983 by M.H. Williams. Adapted by permission.

keep energy intake constant and increase the percentage of carbohydrate calories, a difficult task if you eat high-fat foods.

The other pitfall is that if you are not used to eating a lot of carbohydrates, you could experience diarrhea (especially if increasing your fruits and whole grains).

Meeting Personal Needs

A general rule to ensure optimal carbohydrate intake is to aim for 600 grams of carbohydrates. But this is not very exact. Here's how to figure your personal goals: Aim for 10 grams of carbohydrates for every kilogram you weigh (2.2 pounds = 1 kilogram). For example, if you weigh 125 pounds, you should shoot for 568 grams of carbohydrates.

$$(125/2.2) \times 10 = 568$$

Be aware of the dose-response limit. You will achieve no proportional increase of glycogen storage by eating more carbohydrates than the amount stated above. Consuming beyond the recommended level is like trying to "top off" your car's gas tank after it is full.

One good way to boost your carbohydrate intake is to count grams of carbohydrates. But that is time-consuming. This general plan will get you in a good carbohydrate-loading ballpark:

- Increase your daily grain group servings to 16.
- Increase your nonfat or lowfat dairy servings to 4.
- Increase your fruits and vegetables to 10 servings.

Drinking fruit juices is a fast and easy way to consume carbohydrates. For example, 12 ounces of apple juice provides about 44 grams of carbohydrates. You may want to refer to the list of the top 15 high-carbohydrate foods in chapter 22.

Carbohydrate Sports Drink

For events lasting longer than 90 minutes, a sports drink with a 5-10% carbohydrate solution may improve performance. See Table 16.4 for a sports drink comparison.

PUMPING PROTEIN

Many muscle-building athletes or fitness buffs try to hasten muscle bulking by eating large amounts of protein or supplementing their

Table 16.4   Sports Drinks Compared

Sports drink	Main ingredients	Recommended concentration (%)	Sodium[a] (mg)	Other electrolytes[a]	Calories[a]
Body Fuel 450	Glucose polymers Fructose	4.0	80	20 mg potassium	40
Carbo Plus	Glucose polymers	16.0	5	100 mg potassium 100 mg magnesium	170
Exceed—Fluid Replacement and Energy Drink	Glucose polymers (Polycose brand) Fructose	7.2	66	56 mg potassium	68
Gatorade	Sucrose Glucose	6.0	110	25 mg potassium	50
Gookinaid E.R.G.	Glucose	5.7	70	100 mg potassium	45
Max	Glucose polymers	7.5	15	None	70
Pripps Pluss	Sucrose	7.4	65	Potassium, amount n/a	70
Tour De France Carboplex II	Glucose polymers Fructose	5.9	3	None	45

[a]Per 8-oz serving.

Note. From Coleman, Ellen (1988). *Eating for Endurance.* Palo Alto, CA: Bull Publishing Company. Used with permission of Bull Publishing.

diet with amino acids. Unfortunately, there is no nutritional shortcut to building muscles. You must do it the hard way: Earn your muscles through exercise. Only exercise stimulates muscle growth and strength.

Ironically, the group of athletes shown to consistently have the highest protein needs are endurance athletes, not body builders! The current thinking behind this is that the endurance athlete uses the body's amino acids as an energy source when glycogen stores run out. Fortunately, these amino acids are easily replaced; as study after study has shown, getting protein in the diet is easy to do.

If protein alone would truly aid in building muscles, then a lot of people would look like Mr. and Ms. Olympia with bulging muscles. The average person in the United States eats twice the RDA for protein. Consider that if just an extra 10 grams of protein daily (such as one cup of yogurt) were converted to muscle, you would have 32 pounds of new lean muscle mass by the end of one year. But muscle bulking does not work this way.

Chances are, you're getting more than enough protein to support new muscle growth. Muscle is made up of 22% protein and 70% water. Therefore, one pound of muscle contains only 3-1/2 ounces of protein. As you can see, muscle is mainly water! Excess protein eaten is simply converted to fat, not muscle (or in some cases, excess protein is used as an expensive energy source).

Amino Acids

Likewise, amino acid supplements offer no advantage; they are simply expensive sources of protein. Essential amino acids are conserved wonderfully by the body—they are recycled an average of eight times! Free-form amino acids do not exist in nature. They are processed by cultivation of bacteria, whose amino acid linkages are subsequently treated with enzymatic digestions. Such substances are hardly natural. Amino acid supplements may impair protein metabolism. For example, taking the essential amino acid leucine can inhibit isoleucine metabolism, another essential amino acid.

Side Effects

One possible side effect of high-protein diets is dehydration. To metabolize the excess protein, the body must eliminate its potentially toxic waste product, urea, via the urine. This process requires approximately 1/5 cup of water for every gram of urea excreted. Therefore, extra water loss naturally occurs when you eat more protein than your body needs.

High protein intake also increases calcium excretion, resulting in the elimination of calcium from the body (in the urine). The long-term effects of this reaction are not known, but some researchers warn that it could decrease the bone calcium content, putting you at higher risk for osteoporosis.

Finally, the 1989 *Diet and Health Report* (previously discussed in chapter 13), recommends that protein consumption not exceed twice the RDA for optimal health. Athletes may indeed need a little more protein, but the exact level has yet to be determined. Study after study has shown that athletes consume plenty of protein to meet their athletic needs.

FLUIDS

Water is the nutrient that athletes neglect the most. This forgotten nutrient is essential to life and to performance. It is so abundant, cheap, and readily available that its importance is frequently taken for granted.

Losses of body water amounting to as little as 2% of body weight can significantly impair performance. Yet without making conscious efforts to drink water, you could suffer fluid deficits amounting to 3% before you feel thirsty.

By the time you do feel thirsty, dehydration has most likely set in, partly because the thirst response is blunted during physical exercise. Additionally, many studies have shown that, when given the opportunity, athletes do not drink enough to replace the water lost. Drinking one half to one cup of fluids every 10 to 15 minutes helps prevent dehydration.

Trying to drink while competing—without getting water up your nose—can be an art in itself. One very simple and inexpensive way to overcome this problem is to use a paper cup with a lid and a straw. You can easily get these from a fast-food restaurant, many times at no charge.

You should at the very minimum consume 8 cups of water a day. In addition, monitor your weight before and after training to find out how much water you lost through sweat. Two cups of water weighs one pound. Therefore, you should drink 2 cups of water for every pound lost. For example, if you weighed 150 pounds before workout and 148 pounds after, you should drink 4 cups of water to replace your fluid deficit.

ERGOGENIC AIDS: FOUNTAIN OF HOPE

Many athletes and fitness enthusiasts have searched for that magic pill or supplement that offers that "extra edge," be it quick recovery time or increased energy or strength. These "miracle" substances are referred to as ergogenic aids. By definition, an ergogenic aid is something that can increase the ability to do work.

During my competitive running days (before I was in the nutrition field), I tried all kinds of nutritional aids from wheat germ to dextrose tablets. I once had a well-meaning coach tell me that I should take enough wheat germ that if my veins were cut, I'd bleed wheat germ.

To date no nutritional supplement has been proven to increase performance or give you the winning edge (unless you count carbohydrate sports drinks or carbohydrate loading). Caffeine looks the most promising for enhancing endurance performance, but it also may have side effects that could hamper performance rather than improve it. Caffeine is considered a drug and is banned in the Olympics. However, you would have to drink about 20 cups of coffee to consume the illegal drug level of caffeine, and benefits to performance have been seen at the level equal to only 2-1/2 cups of coffee.

Many of the products sold to increase performance—such as carnitine or bee pollen—are useless. Why are they sold? Money. Many of the claims for ergogenic aids are made by the companies that sell them. They are motivated by profit, and often they will pay athletes to endorse their products.

The following story illustrates a good example of this profit motive. My husband, Jeff, owns a couple of running stores. Salespeople come in at least twice a month pushing some nutritional supplement. They try to convince Jeff to carry their products because the products are "great for repeat sales and moneymakers," not because they benefit athletes. Indeed, Jeff could generate extra revenue by carrying these products. However, he refuses to sell them for ethical reasons—these supplements have no demonstrated merit.

Placebo Effect

Sometimes an athlete believes so strongly in a supplement that an inert substance such as a sugar pill will work. This reaction is known as a placebo effect, or the power of belief. The performance benefit results from this placebo phenomenon, not from the actual supplement.

Athletes also may believe a nutritional aid works because of coincidence, or what I call the "lucky underwear syndrome." For example, an athlete may feel that he or she has to wear the exact same underwear that was worn during his or her best performance. Likewise, an athlete may have broken a record on the same day that he or she took honey and erroneously believes that honey was responsible. In reality, of course, the success resulted from hard training combined with other factors.

Vitamin and Mineral Supplements

Everyone agrees that a nutrient deficiency will hurt athletic performance. Several studies have shown, however, that supplementing vitamins and minerals beyond the Recommended Dietary Allowance does not improve performance unless a deficiency existed in the first place. Furthermore, using megadoses of nutrients, especially singular nutrient supplementations, can be dangerous (as discussed in chapter 14). But performance can also suffer from megadosing. For example, large doses of niacin can inhibit fat from being transported from storage to exercising muscle. As a result, the muscle relies more on glycogen, which could cause glycogen to be depleted at a quicker rate and fatigue to hit sooner. See Table 16.5 for a review and summary of ergogenic aids and performance.

Table 16.5   Nutritional Ergogenic Aids

Supplement	Demonstrated benefits	Possible negative consequences
Amino acids/protein	–	1. Metabolic imbalance from single amino acids 2. Excess stored as fat 3. Dehydration 4. Increases calcium loss
B-complex vitamins	–	1. Nerve damage
Bee pollen	–	1. Allergic reaction
Caffeine	+/–	1. Diarrhea 2. Rapid pulse 3. Dehydration 4. Gastric distress
Carnitine	–	?
Honey	–	1. Rebound hypoglycemia

(Cont.)

Table 16.5 (Continued)

Supplement	Demonstrated benefits	Possible negative consequences
Niacin	–	1. Slows fat mobilization 2. Increases glycogen loss
Octacosonal	–	?
Ornithine/arginine	–	1. See "Amino acids"
Riboflavin	?	?
Royal bee jelly	–	?
Salt tablets	–	1. Intracellular dehydration
Sodium bicarbonate	–	1. Diarrhea 2. Alkalosis
Vitamin C	?	1. Diarrhea 2. Impairs copper absorption 3. Interferes with B-12 metabolism
Vitamin E	–	1. Diarrhea 2. Muscle weakness
Wheat germ/wheat germ oil	–	?

– = no demonstrated benefit; + = benefit; ? = unknown or questionable.

Note. Based on information from American Dietetic Association, 1986.

CHAPTER

17

Time Management for Meals: Meals in a Hurry

"My idea of time management for meals is pushing a microwave button."—

insurance agent

I have clients embarrassed to admit that they don't cook. I know few people who relish the thought of coming home and having to make dinner after putting in a full workday. For some people, even the thought of cooking makes them feel exhausted. But preparing dinner doesn't have to be a big production. Remember, you don't have to have hot-cooked meals to enjoy good nutrition. In this chapter, I will share timesaving measures to get your meals prepared in a flash, so you can have more time to enjoy your evening.

As you learned in chapter 2, successful eating on the run begins with planning. It's important—especially when you know you will be home for dinner the upcoming week—to plan some meals ahead of time and to have ingredients on hand. This alone will save gobs of time and spare you the experience of staring at the cupboards waiting for divine inspiration, night after night.

In this chapter we will focus on the other keys to getting you out of the kitchen faster: organization, utilizing pre-prepped food, planned-overs, and timesaving gadgets.

BASIC ORGANIZATION

How would you categorize your cupboards and refrigerator?

	____ Disaster area
	____ Organized mess
	____ Creatures from the black lagoon
	____ "Let's Make a Deal" (or what's behind pantry door number 2?)
	____ Room for improvement

Kitchen storage space seems to be a problem in most homes. Just as the amount of time it takes to complete a task expands to fill the time allotted for it, your kitchen supplies expand to fill kitchen storage space. If you increase storage space but fail to organize it, you could end up with a bigger mess.

When you do not know where an item is, you waste valuable time hunting for it. And you may suffer mental anguish from the search. The answer to avoiding these frustrating scavenger hunts lies in organization.

Some ideas for arranging kitchen storage areas are listed below. The basic principle here is to group together items that will be used together—it's similar to the way that grocery stores are arranged. Try implementing the ideas that will save you time.

Cupboards.

1. Keep frequently used items within easy reach.
2. Alphabetize your spices for speedy identification or use a spice-rack organizer.
3. Store utensils and foods near the areas you'll use them most often (pot holders next to oven, pans by the stove).
4. Store foods so that the labels are facing you, so you can easily identify them.
5. Group your foods for easy locating:

- bottled items
- canned items
- dry foods
- grains
- packaged foods
- paper goods

6. Consider installing a "step-up" shelf (a shelf half the usual width or less placed between two other shelves) for small items:

- cups
- saucers
- small dishes
- spices

7. Have a separate storage area for these bigger pieces:

- appliances
- gadgets
- mixing bowls
- pots and pans

Drawers.

1. Eliminate any junk or clutter.
2. Partition drawers for storage of utensils:

- baking utensils (measuring devices and so on)
- eating utensils
- gadgets
- knives
- stove-top utensils

Counter Top.

1. Store these regularly used appliances ready-to-go on the counter:

- blender
- can opener
- food processor
- mixer
- toaster

2. Place food staples in canisters on the counter to save time digging them out of drawers and cabinets.

- beans
- bread (in bread box)
- flour
- noodles

- rice
- other

3. Place grazing foods ready-to-go in a basket.
4. If feasible, hang gadgets, utensils, or pots on the wall closest to where you use them.

Refrigerator.

1. Take advantage of preorganized areas:
   - margarine keeper
   - meat/cheese keeper
   - side-door storage
   - vegetable/fruit drawer
2. Store foods in easy-to-see, ready-to-use containers:
   - clear jars
   - transparent dishes
3. Keep frequently used items in spots that are easy to reach.
4. Divide your refrigerator space into four areas for the following categories of foods:
   - beverages
   - dairy
   - produce
   - proteins (meats, cheese, tofu)
     (FAST TIP: Also have a separate area for leftovers.)
5. Use the FIFO (first in, first out) principle. This will help to prevent these inefficiencies:
   - waste
   - re-buying the same food (duplicate buildup)
   - multiple containers of the same food

PRE-PREPARATION

Pre-preparation steps often seem as if you are going back one step to move ahead two. For example, chopping, slicing, and dicing food can be time-consuming and boring. Such tasks often present the most obstacles when deciding what to eat.

The more rungs you eliminate on the food-preparation ladder, the more time you have to enjoy. Having food pre-prepped or ready-to-go when you need it is essential for grazers. Pre-prepped food also makes it easier to throw together an evening meal when you feel drained after a hard day. Here are some ideas to get you quickly through this task.

Buy It Pre-Prepped

Instead of slicing and dicing your knuckles to the bone, consider buying your food in the least time-consuming form. I can think of no better example than grated cheese. You can now buy lowfat cheese grated. So not only do you save prep time, but you don't have to clean the cheese grater!

You can buy your turkey sliced, onions chopped, garlic minced, and so forth. Many grocery stores are packaging produce that is washed and ready-to-go. You can take advantage of the salad bars that are also popping up in grocery stores and buy produce ready-to-eat.

The only disadvantage of buying food already prepped is the added cost. I think it's worth it. You may actually save money when you compare what your time is worth. List 17.1 gives you a timesaving grocery list.

Pre-Prep Food Yourself

Doing it yourself is a good option, especially if you are watching your pennies. The best technique is to prepare all the food at one time,

List 17.1
Timesavers from the Grocery Store

Meats
  Boneless, skinless chicken
  Diced chicken
  Ground turkey
  Turkey breast, cubed or sliced

Canned (preferably no added salt)
  Beans
    black
    garbanzo
    kidney
    pinto

Dairy
  Cheese (lowfat varieties)
    cubed, grated, sliced
    single-serving size

Produce
  Cherry tomatoes (instead of whole tomatoes)
  Chopped cabbage
  Chopped garlic (in a jar)
  Chopped lettuce
  Chopped onion
  Salad bar produce
  Sliced green peppers
  Sliced mushrooms

which will save you time in the long run and make the food readily available. A food processor will save you even more time. Otherwise, a good sharp knife will do.

Ready, set, go. Set aside a time for batch chopping, slicing, and dicing. You might want to consider doing it right after grocery shopping before you put the food away.

Next, use the Baggie method of food control, in which items such as vegetables are divided into plastic bags for convenient storage and easy accessibility. Clear storage bowls will also do the trick. With everything sliced and ready-to-go, you can put together a meal in a hurry.

TAKE ADVANTAGE OF COOKING MOMENTS: PLANNED-OVERS

Planned-overs are intentional leftovers, like pre-prepping an entire meal. With this technique, also known as batch cooking, you can take advantage of your cooking moments.

Essentially you double or even triple your favorite recipe. By doing this, you can prepare multiple meals in the same amount of time as it takes to fix one. Then you have an instant home-cooked meal ready-to-eat in a jiffy, usually just a zap away.

Or planned-overs can simply be cooking a few extra chicken breasts or meats, and freezing them for later. Here's how to make the most of planned-overs:

1. Divide your individual meals into freezer containers to make your own TV dinners. This method will also help preserve nutrients because you won't be reheating the same batch of food several times.
2. Recycle the compartmentalized plates from commercial frozen dinners. Use them to ''pre-plate'' and freeze your planned-overs.
3. Store meals in containers in which they can be reheated. If you use a microwave, be sure your container is microwave-proof.
4. Stagger your planned-overs to prevent burnout.
5. Label and date your planned-overs, or it is easy to forget what's in the container and when it was made.
6. For a cook-free workweek with home-style food, make meals ahead on the weekend.

TIMESAVING GADGETS

Here are a few gadgets worth investing in. Of course, gadgets will only save time if you use them; otherwise they can become obstacles of clutter. Pick and choose what would help you.

Cordless Mixer.   It's always ready-to-go when mounted on the wall with all of its attachments. There's no hassle searching for your regular mixer and its extension cord and beaters. Also, you are not confined to being near an electric outlet.

Crockpot: Throw and Go.   The nice thing about Crockpots is you just throw together a few choice ingredients, set the thermostat, and it's off to work (or wherever) you go. You arrive home to a hot-cooked meal without slaving over a hot stove. Some all-in-one meals that work well with Crockpots are stewed chicken, soups, and beans (split pea, lentils, black bean).

Tips: A Crockpot cooks more efficiently when it is half full. When adapting your favorite recipes, you'll need less liquid. This is because the fluid doesn't evaporate (the lid is left on during cooking).

Garlic Press.   If you love fresh garlic flavor, a garlic press is the fastest way to get minced garlic. One squish through this little press and you have minced garlic, without the traditional tedious chopping.

Kitchen Shears.   I finally broke down and bought a pair of these, and it has really simplified irksome tasks such as snipping parsley or chives. Many food packages also need to be cut open, and kitchen scissors do a quick job here.

Food Processor.   Don't tell me. You received one for Christmas but still haven't gotten around to using it. Solution: Keep it on your counter ready to go (this means attachments nearby). It will save a lot of time.

Microwave (of course).   If you are 1 of the 2 out of 10 people who do *not* own a microwave, you are missing out on one of the most timesaving appliances of all. Here are a few things a microwave can do in a matter of seconds:

- Reheat care packages given by loved ones
- Defrost in a pinch
- Reheat leftovers and planned-overs
- Quickly melt lowfat cheese on tortillas, bagels, crackers, or vegetables
- Heat frozen-packed vegetables
- Boil water

Microwaves can also be used for "full cooking," such as baking a potato in a matter of only minutes, cooking chicken and fish, and so on. Microwave cooking also retains more nutrients than traditional cooking. And one of the things I like best about microwave cooking is that it usually means less mess (fewer dishes to clean).

TEN TIMESAVING HABITS

Get into the practices listed below, and your tour of duty in the kitchen will be much quicker.

1. Assemble all ingredients, utensils, and pans before you begin cooking. This allows for an efficient cooking effort without having to stop and search.
2. To keep dishes to a minimum (and save time cleaning them), try these tips:
   - Mix everything in a large measuring cup instead of a mixing bowl.
   - Stir ingredients with a measuring spoon instead of a big spoon.
   - Use cooking/baking dishes that will double as serving dishes.
   - Use a divided skillet to prepare more than one item.
3. Make use of your downtime. For example, set the table while waiting for the microwave.
4. Quickly keep track of foods and other essentials that need to be replaced so that you don't have to suddenly run out to the store. Keep a pad and pen near cupboards, or a magnetic board or chalkboard in your kitchen.
5. Take advantage of buffet-style fixings (everyone assembles their own meal), such as chicken tacos, deli night, or home-style salad bar.
6. For easy salads, make a large batch of salad and store in an airtight container (no dressing or spices). This will keep your salad fresh and crisp for 2 to 3 days.
7. Use fresh pasta (from deli section) rather than dried. It will save you considerable cooking time. And the flavor is fresher.
8. Stockpile staples. Make sure you have an ample supply of routinely used food items.
9. Take advantage of one-dish meals (aka casseroles) and one-minute meals listed in the next chapter.
10. Plan. Plan. Plan.

For specific quick meal ideas, the next three chapters will provide recipes for quick, easy meals and meals that can be made in 60 seconds or less, seven basic meals, and the ultimate no-work 7-day eating on the run menu.

CHAPTER

18

Quick: Easy Meals to Throw Together

"Cook? What's that?"—

single real estate agent

This chapter includes meals that are quick and easy to prepare. These meals are staples in my house because they easily can be cooked in large quantities for planned-overs.

You will find pasta sauces listed here. This may seem surprising since pasta dishes traditionally take a long time to prepare. However, the availability of deli-fresh pastas facilitates the preparation of sumptuous pasta meals in a flash. For example, angel hair pasta takes only 60 seconds to cook in boiling water! All you have to do is vary the sauce for another quick meal.

Here are the recipes found in this chapter:

1. *Quick Marinara Sauce.* The carrots in this sauce boost the vitamin A value and contribute to a thick, hearty sauce.
2. *Spinach Cheese Pasta.* This is one of my daughter's favorite meals!
3. *Turkey Chili.* This is great for leftovers.
4. *Relax-While-It-Cooks Foil Chicken.* This all-in-one meal is the poultry equivalent of a pot-roast meal.

5. *Tostadas.* These tostadas are much lower in fat than the traditional versions because the tortillas are not fried, but rather are oven-crisped.
6. *Oregano Chicken Soup.* This easy comfort food will soothe you on mind-bustling days. This recipe makes plenty of home-cooked soup for a couple of meals.
7. *Make-Ahead Stuffed Potatoes.* This is one of my favorite recipes. They taste good and can be made in large batches so that one effort will save oodles of time in the future. Add this recipe to your cookathon days.
8. *Mexican Stir Fry.* The beauty of this meal is that it is all in one skillet and can be made with any type of meat: lean beef, turkey tenderloin, chicken, shrimp.
9. *Breakfast Bars.* This make-ahead breakfast tastes so good that you might want to eat it as a snack or dessert. It was adapted from a Grape-Nuts recipe. My favorite fruits to use are boysenberries and raspberries.

RECIPES

QUICK MARINARA SAUCE
(serves 4)

Olive Oil Pam
Chopped garlic (2 fresh cloves, or 2 teaspoons
  from jar)
1 teaspoon dried oregano, crushed
Dash basil
1 carrot, finely grated
28-oz can chopped stewed tomatoes
1/2 small can tomato paste (or 1/3 cup)
9-oz pkg. fresh angel hair pasta, cooked

NUTRITION (per serving):	
Calories:	412
Fat:	1 gram
% Fat calories:	2

Spray large skillet with Pam. Add garlic, oregano, basil, and carrot. Sauté carrot. Add stewed tomatoes and tomato paste. Simmer about 5 minutes. Pour over pasta.

Timesaver Tip: Double the sauce, toss one portion with the hot pasta, and freeze for a future meal.

SPINACH CHEESE PASTA
(serves 4)

Olive Oil Pam
2 cloves of garlic (or equivalent in garlic
  powder)
10-oz pkg. frozen chopped spinach, thawed
  and drained
1 cup lowfat cottage cheese
1/2 cup grated Parmesan cheese
9-oz pkg. fresh angel hair pasta, cooked

NUTRITION (per serving):	
Calories:	302
Fat:	6 grams
% Fat calories:	18

Spray large skillet with Pam and sauté garlic. Add spinach. Next add cheeses and stir thoroughly until cheese is melted. Stir in pasta.

Timesaver Tip: Put spinach in refrigerator to thaw before you go to work in the morning.

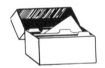

TURKEY CHILI
(serves 10)

1 lb ground turkey
1 large onion, chopped
3 16-oz cans pinto or kidney beans
28-oz can chopped, stewed tomatoes
1 tablespoon chili powder
1 tablespoon cumin powder
1/2 jar of salsa (about 1/2 cup)
Lowfat grated cheddar cheese (optional)

NUTRITION (per serving):	
Calories:	228
Fat:	6 grams
% Fat calories:	24

In a large pot, brown turkey with chopped onion. Add beans, tomatoes, seasonings, and salsa. Cook until hot. If desired, garnish with cheese.

Timesaver Tip: Open cans while turkey is browning. Buy frozen chopped onions.

RELAX-WHILE-IT-COOKS FOIL CHICKEN
(serves 4)

1 cup barbecue sauce
4 skinless chicken breasts
1 green pepper, sliced
2 carrots, diagonally cut or cut into strips
2 small potatoes, thinly sliced

NUTRITION (per serving):	
Calories:	263
Fat:	4 grams
% Fat calories:	15

Preheat oven to 350°. Line cookie sheet with aluminum foil. Pour 1/2 cup of barbecue sauce, and place chicken on top of sauce. Pour the remainder of barbecue sauce on top of chicken. Add the cut vegetables. Add another layer of aluminum foil, and join with bottom foil to fold sides together. Bake about 35 minutes (until pink tinge is gone inside chicken).

Timesaver Tip: Buy boneless, skinless chicken breasts. Make additional chicken breasts for a next-day barbecue chicken sandwich. Don't worry about exact measurements—the eyeball technique works just fine here.

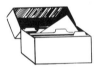

TOSTADAS
(makes 3 servings of 2 tostadas each)

6 corn tortillas
1 can pinto beans or vegetarian refried beans
1/2 head of lettuce, shredded
1 cup lowfat cheddar cheese, grated
1/2 cup chopped, stewed tomatoes
Salsa (optional)
Cilantro, snipped (optional)

NUTRITION (per serving):	
Calories:	354
Fat:	10 grams
% Fat calories:	24

(This data is based on vegetarian refried beans—plain pinto beans would have a lower fat content.)

Preheat oven to 350°. Place corn tortillas on oven shelf and bake until light brown (about 7 minutes). Layer the remaining ingredients in the following order (according to your liking): beans, lettuce, tomatoes, salsa, and a hint of cilantro. Top with cheese.

Timesaver Tip: While tortillas are crispening in the oven, prepare garnishes. Have everyone assemble their own tostada for personal taste and further timesaving.

OREGANO CHICKEN SOUP
(serves 6 large portions)

6 cups water
1 tablespoon oregano
1/2 teaspoon celery seed
1 teaspoon onion powder
3 chicken breasts, skinless, boneless
28-oz can chopped, stewed tomatoes, including
  juice
2 carrots, sliced
1 cup dark green leafy vegetable, chopped
  (spinach, Swiss chard, leeks, bok choy)

NUTRITION (per serving):	
Calories:	123
Fat:	2 grams
% Fat calories:	15

Stove-top Method: In 5-quart pot (or Dutch oven) combine all ingredients. Simmer until chicken is done. Remove chicken and cut or shred it into bite-size pieces. Place chicken bites back into pot. Soup's ready!

Crockpot Method: Reduce water to 5 cups. Combine all ingredients. Place in Crockpot, cover, and cook on low 7 to 9 hours. Dinner will be ready when you arrive home. Yum!

Timesaver Tip: Use dried spices, rather than chopping their fresh counterparts (celery, onion, garlic). Use boneless, skinless chicken breasts for hassle-free soup. Throw in an extra breast or two, and you'll have ready-cooked chicken for another meal. For the easiest method, use a Crockpot.

MAKE-AHEAD STUFFED POTATOES
(serves 4)

4 medium potatoes
1/2 cup nonfat yogurt
1 pint lowfat cottage cheese
1 cup lowfat cheddar cheese

NUTRITION (per serving):	
Calories:	322
Fat:	6 grams
% Fat calories:	17

Pierce potatoes, and microwave until done (about 13 to 16 minutes) for the four potatoes. Cut potatoes in half, and scoop out each potato, leaving a thin shell. Using either a food processor or a mixer, blend potato scoopings, yogurt, and cottage cheese. Refill potato shells with potato-pulp mixture. Top with grated cheese. Broil in conventional oven until cheese is melted.

Timesaver Tip: Make ahead and freeze. Eat one for breakfast, lunch, or dinner.

MEXICAN STIR FRY—AKA FAJITAS
(serves 4)

2 tablespoons fat-free Italian dressing
2 tablespoons lime or lemon juice
1 medium onion, thinly sliced into long strips
  or rings
2 medium red or green peppers, cut into thin
  strips
1 lb of lean meat, chopped (turkey, skinless
  chicken, or extra lean beef such as round
  steak)
1 medium tomato, chopped
1/2 cup cilantro, snipped
Grated lowfat cheese (optional)
Salsa (optional)

NUTRITION (per serving):	
Calories:	322
Fat:	6 grams
% Fat calories:	17

In large skillet add fat-free dressing and lime juice. Cook and stir onion strips for 1-1/2 minutes. Add peppers, cook, and stir until crispy tender (about 1 minute). Add meat; cook and stir until done (about 2 to 3 minutes). Add chopped tomato and cilantro. Cook and stir for about another minute. Serve with whole wheat tortillas. Garnish if desired with salsa and cheese.

Timesaver Tip: Purchase turkey tidbits, fresh turkey breast/tenderloin precut into bite-size pieces.

BREAKFAST BARS
(serves 8)

2-1/2 cups Grape-Nuts
3 tablespoons honey
2 8-oz containers nonfat fruit yogurt
1 cup fruit
2/3 cup nonfat dry milk

NUTRITION (per serving):	
Calories:	224
Fat:	trace
% Fat calories:	0

Spray a square pan (about 8 in. × 8 in.) with vegetable cooking spray. Line pan with about 3/4 cup Grape-Nuts. In a blender combine honey, yogurt, fruit, and nonfat dry milk. Blend until smooth. Fold in 1 cup Grape-Nuts. Pour yogurt mixture into pan. Top with remaining 3/4 cup Grape-Nuts. Freeze for at least 4 hours. Cut into rectangles (they will look like ice-cream sandwiches).

Timesaver Tip: Keep extra on hand frozen, so it is always ready.

19

Quickest: One-Minute Meals

Can you squeeze just one minute into your busy schedule? All too often I have heard, "I don't have time to make breakfast (lunch, dinner)." That's why I developed the one-minute meal concept. This chapter has 16 new additional recipes (a total of 40) to choose from.

Sixty seconds or less is all it will take to make a healthy mini-meal. The ol' "I don't have time" excuse is no longer true.

The speediest one-minute meal is the Quickie, designed for breakneck nutrition survival when you are in a negative time crunch. The Quickie is simply a glass of nonfat milk followed by an orange juice chaser; it takes all of 19 seconds to prepare. This combination may not seem ideal, but it supplies about 30% of daily calcium needs and 162% of daily vitamin C requirements. You can do that!

I have developed and time-tested these mini-meals to make sure that they can indeed be made in under 60 seconds. And, of course, they do taste good, too! For additional nutritional value, you may want to combine these mini-meals with grazing snacks listed in chapter 2.

Don't worry about measuring the ingredients. The eyeball technique ("it looks like a cup") will suffice. The measurements are there as a guide, but they also serve as the basis for the nutritional information provided.

Remember, have all ingredients assembled so you can speed through these recipes. The preparation time is based on ingredients purchased in the form they are called for. For example, the cheese is bought grated. You certainly can grate your own; it just requires a little more time.

Here is a list of the one-minute meal recipes that follow:

- Tropical Wake-Up Smoothie
- Hula Bagel
- Stuffed Cantaloupe
- Bagel Melt
- Banana Roll-Up
- Zippy Turkey Hoagie
- Submarine Cheese Melt
- Lox and Bagel
- Pita Chili Melt
- Savory Chick-Pea Spread (Hummus) and Pita
- Tortilla Pinwheels
- Peanut Butter Banana Shake
- Mini-Gouda and Baguette
- Greek Stuffed Pita
- Mexican Pita Pizza
- Peach Smoothie
- The Quickie
- English Muffin Melt
- Curried Chicken Celery
- Pita Surprise
- Ak-Mak and Cheese
- Turkey Roll-Up
- Cottage Cheese Delight
- Orange Reveille
- Tortilla Sandwich
- Basic Sandwich
- Pita Salad
- Quesadilla
- Cereal and Milk
- Turkey Bagel
- Banana Health Shake
- Rice Cake Crunch
- Strawberry Yogurt Frappé

- Quick Pizza
- Pita Pan
- Fiesta Bean Burrito
- Peanut Butter Melt
- Abba Zabba
- Cottage Raisin Toast
- Tuna Salad Pita

ONE-MINUTE MEAL RECIPES

TROPICAL WAKE-UP SMOOTHIE
Prep time: 50 seconds

1/2 cup frozen fruit (banana, pineapple, or peach)
1 cup nonfat yogurt (tropical flavor)
1/4 cup orange juice

NUTRITION (per serving):	
Calories:	209
Fat:	trace
% Fat calories	0

Mix all ingredients in a blender until smooth.

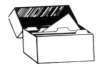

HULA BAGEL
Prep time: 46 seconds

1 bagel, sliced
1/3 cup lowfat ricotta cheese
1/4 cup crushed pineapple, drained
Dash of nutmeg

NUTRITION (per serving):	
Calories:	250
Fat:	5 grams
% Fat calories:	18

1. Combine ricotta cheese, crushed pineapple, and nutmeg.
2. Spread mixture on bagel slices.

STUFFED CANTALOUPE
Prep time: 25 seconds

1/2 cantaloupe
1/2 cup nonfat cottage cheese
Dash of cinnamon

NUTRITION (per serving):	
Calories:	139
Fat:	0 grams
% Fat calories:	0

1. Scoop cottage cheese into hollow section of cantaloupe. 2. Sprinkle with cinnamon.

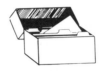

BAGEL MELT
Prep time: 54 seconds

1 bagel sliced
2 slices lowfat American cheese

NUTRITION (per serving):	
Calories:	233
Fat:	5 grams
% Fat calories:	21

1. Place cheese between bagel halves. 2. Microwave until melted.

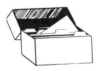

BANANA ROLL-UP
Prep time: 60 seconds

1/2 banana
2 teaspoons natural-style peanut butter
1 teaspoon honey
1 tablespoon wheat germ
2 tablespoons nugget-type cereal
1 teaspoon allspice or pumpkin spice

NUTRITION (per serving):	
Calories:	199
Fat:	6 grams
% Fat calories:	25

1. Spread peanut butter on banana until covered. 2. Drizzle honey over banana and peanut butter. 3. Mix wheat germ, nugget cereal, and allspice together. 4. Roll the peanut butter covered banana in the wheat germ mix.

ZIPPY TURKEY HOAGIE
Prep time: 35 seconds

1 deli-style roll 2 tablespoons fat-free Italian dressing 1 slice deli turkey breast (about 1 oz) 1 oz lowfat cheese Green leaf lettuce	**NUTRITION** (per serving): Calories: 197 Fat: 5 grams % Fat calories: 20

1. Spread fat-free dressing on roll. 2. Layer turkey and cheese. 3. Add lettuce.

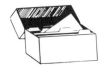

SUBMARINE CHEESE MELT
Prep time: 59 seconds

1 deli-style roll 2 tablespoons fat-free Italian dressing 1 oz lowfat American cheese 1 oz lowfat Swiss cheese Green leaf lettuce, shredded 1/4 tomato, sliced	**NUTRITION** (per serving): Calories: 312 Fat: 6 grams % Fat calories: 17

1. Open roll into an open-faced butterfly. 2. Spread dressing. 3. Add cheese on each part of the roll. 4. Microwave until cheese starts to melt. While microwaving, chop lettuce and tomato. 5. Add the lettuce and tomato to cheese melt. Note: This is one of my favorites.

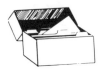

LOX AND BAGEL
Prep time: 47 seconds

1 whole bagel, sliced 1 oz lox or smoked salmon 1 oz ultra-lowfat ricotta cheese	**NUTRITION** (per serving): Calories: 196 Fat: 3 grams % Fat calories 12

Spread ricotta cheese on bagel and add lox.

PITA CHILI MELT
Prep time: 59 seconds

1/2 large whole wheat pita bread
1/2 cup canned pinto beans
2 tablespoons grated lowfat cheddar cheese
1 tablespoon diced green chili

NUTRITION (per serving):	
Calories:	359
Fat:	4 grams
% Fat calories:	10

1. Put beans, cheese, and chili into pita bread. 2. Microwave until cheese melts.

SAVORY CHICK-PEA SPREAD (HUMMUS) AND PITA
Prep time: 58 seconds

1 can (15-1/2 oz) chick-peas (save the 1/4 cup liquid)
1 tablespoon lemon juice (fresh or bottled)
1/4 teaspoon garlic powder
2 tablespoons tahini (sesame paste) or sesame seeds
1 small pita bread

NUTRITION (per serving):	
Calories:	278
Fat:	4 grams
% Fat calories:	14

1. In a blender or food processor, puree first four ingredients until smooth. 2. While chick-peas are blending, cut pita bread into triangles. 3. Serve hummus as a dip or spread. (1 serving = 1 pita bread and 1/4 cup hummus.)

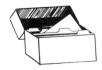

TORTILLA PINWHEELS
Prep time: 48 seconds

2 leaves green leaf lettuce
2 thinly sliced pieces of deli-cut turkey
1/2 sliced tomato
1 whole wheat tortilla

NUTRITION (per serving):	
Calories:	201
Fat:	5 grams
% Fat calories:	22

1. Place lettuce on tortilla. 2. Add turkey for the next layer, followed by the sliced tomato. 3. Roll up like a burrito. 4. Insert 4 toothpicks to prevent from unrolling. Then slice into 4 pinwheels (each will have a toothpick). Note: This elegant but simple recipe can also be used for quick appetizers.

PEANUT BUTTER BANANA SHAKE
Prep time: 57 seconds

1 cup nonfat milk
1 tablespoon chunky, natural-style peanut
  butter
1 teaspoon vanilla
1 frozen banana (best to freeze in thin slices)

NUTRITION (per serving):	
Calories:	295
Fat:	9 grams
% Fat calories:	27

1. Using blender, blend the milk, frozen banana slices, and vanilla.
2. While blending, add peanut butter. Blend until smooth.

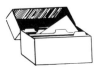

MINI-GOUDA AND BAGUETTE
Prep time: 60 seconds

1 mini reduced-fat Gouda cheese (Mini
  Bonbel)
1 small (6 in.) baguette
2 marinated artichoke hearts, chopped

NUTRITION (per serving):	
Calories:	186
Fat:	6 grams
% Fat calories:	30

1. Slice cheese thinly and place on both halves of bread. 2. Add artichoke hearts. 3. Microwave until slightly melted. Note: This is one of my favorites.

GREEK STUFFED PITA
Prep time: 60 seconds

2 fresh spinach leaves, chopped
2 tablespoons crumbled feta cheese
2 small cubes Laughing Cow reduced cheese
1/2 large pita

NUTRITION (per serving):	
Calories:	259
Fat:	8 grams
% Fat calories:	27

1. Combine spinach and cheeses. 2. Stuff into pita. 3. Melt in microwave.

MEXICAN PITA PIZZA
Prep time: 60 seconds

1 small whole wheat pita
2 tablespoons tomato sauce
1/4 cup canned pinto beans, drained and
    mashed
1 oz mozzarella cheese, grated
Dash oregano

NUTRITION (per serving):	
Calories:	274
Fat:	5 grams
% Fat calories:	18

1. Spread tomato sauce on pita bread. 2. Add pinto beans. 3. Sprinkle with cheese. 4. Top lightly with oregano.

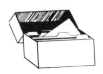

PEACH SMOOTHIE
Prep time: 53 seconds

1 cup frozen, unsweetened peaches
1/2 cup nonfat vanilla or peach yogurt
1/4 cup nonfat milk
1 teaspoon vanilla
Dash nutmeg

NUTRITION (per serving):	
Calories:	324
Fat:	Trace
% Fat calories:	0

Combine all ingredients in blender until smooth.

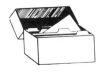

THE QUICKIE
Prep time: 19 seconds

1 cup nonfat milk
1 cup orange juice

NUTRITION (per serving):	
Calories:	198
Fat:	0 grams
% Fat calories	0

1. Pour milk into cup and drink. 2. Pour juice into glass and drink.

ENGLISH MUFFIN MELT
Prep time: 54 seconds

1 wheat English muffin
1 slice lowfat Swiss cheese

NUTRITION (per serving):	
Calories:	211
Fat:	5 grams
% Fat calories:	22

1. Cut English muffin in half. 2. Place 1/2 slice cheese on each muffin. 3. Bake in broiler or microwave oven.

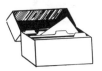

CURRIED CHICKEN CELERY
Prep time: 58 seconds

2 oz chicken, diced, or 1/2 5-oz can of white
   chunk chicken
1/4 teaspoon curry powder
1/2 teaspoon dried mustard powder
1 celery stalk, diced
1 tablespoon lemon juice
2 slices wheat bread

NUTRITION (per serving):	
Calories:	234
Fat:	4 grams
% Fat calories:	15

1. Add lemon juice, celery, and spices to chicken and mix well.
2. Spread on bread.

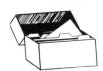

PITA SURPRISE
Prep time: 28 seconds

1/2 large wheat pita bread
1/2 cup leftovers (anything—beans, salad, tur-
   key, etc.)

NUTRITION (per serving):	
Calories:	Variable
Fat:	Variable
% Fat calories:	Variable

Put leftovers in pita.

AK-MAK AND CHEESE
Prep time: 11 seconds

1 oz lowfat cheese
2 to 4 Ak-mak or RyKrisp crackers

NUTRITION (per serving):	
Calories:	100
Fat:	0–4 grams
% Fat calories:	20

Place cheese on crackers.

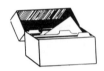

TURKEY ROLL-UP
Prep time: 20 seconds

2 oz sliced turkey
1 carrot stick
1 romaine lettuce leaf

NUTRITION (per serving):	
Calories:	98
Fat:	2 grams
% Fat calories:	18

1. Place turkey on lettuce leaf. 2. Place carrot on top of turkey and roll up.

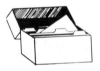

COTTAGE CHEESE DELIGHT
Prep time: 60 seconds

1/2 cup lowfat cottage cheese
2 teaspoons lemon juice
Dash of garlic powder
5 celery sticks
Dash of paprika

NUTRITION (per serving):	
Calories:	97
Fat:	1 gram
% Fat calories:	12

1. Mix all ingredients except celery in blender until smooth. 2. Dip celery into mixture and eat!

ORANGE REVEILLE
Prep time: 59 seconds

6-oz can orange juice concentrate, thawed
2 cans water
1/4 cup nonfat dried milk powder
9 ice cubes
1 teaspoon vanilla

NUTRITION (per serving):	
Calories:	234
Fat:	Trace
% Fat calories:	Trace

1. Mix all ingredients in blender until they reach desired consistency. 2. Yields 2 servings.

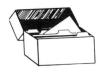

TORTILLA SANDWICH
Prep time: 18 seconds

2 whole wheat tortillas
2 oz chicken (or leftover protein source)
2 lettuce leaves

NUTRITION (per serving):	
Calories:	307
Fat:	7 grams
% Fat calories:	21

Place chicken and lettuce between tortillas.

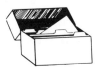

BASIC SANDWICH
Prep time: 21 seconds

2 slices whole wheat bread
2 oz tuna, chicken, turkey, lowfat cheese, or
 other protein source
1 romaine lettuce leaf

NUTRITION (per serving):	
Calories:	225
Fat:	4 grams
% Fat calories:	15

Place ingredients between bread.

PITA SALAD
Prep time: 60 seconds

1/2 large wheat pita bread 1 oz tofu cubes 1/2 cup salad Dash of salad herbs Dash of lemon juice	**NUTRITION** (per serving): **Calories:** 191 **Fat:** 2 grams **% Fat calories:** 11

1. Mix tofu, salad, herbs, and lemon juice. 2. Place mixture in pita bread.

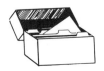

QUESADILLA
Prep time: 58 seconds

1 oz lowfat cheddar cheese, grated or sliced 1 tablespoon salsa 1 teaspoon cilantro 1 whole wheat tortilla	**NUTRITION** (per serving): **Calories:** 182 **Fat:** 6 grams **% Fat calories:** 29

1. Place cheese, salsa, and cilantro on tortilla. 2. Heat until melted in microwave or broiler.

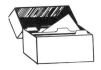

CEREAL AND MILK
Prep time: 31 seconds

1/2 to 1 cup whole grain cereal 1/2 to 1 cup nonfat milk 5 strawberries or 1/2 banana, sliced	**NUTRITION** (per serving): **Calories:** 196 **Fat:** Trace **% Fat calories:** Trace

Place ingredients in bowl.

TURKEY BAGEL
Prep time: 41 seconds

2 oz sliced turkey breast
1 whole wheat bagel
1 leaf romaine lettuce

NUTRITION (per serving):	
Calories:	270
Fat:	3 grams
% Fat calories:	10

1. Slice bagel. 2. Add turkey and lettuce.

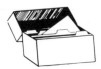

BANANA HEALTH SHAKE
Prep time: 60 seconds

1 whole ripe banana
1/4 cup nonfat dried milk powder
1/2 cup orange juice
1 teaspoon vanilla
Dash of nutmeg
5 ice cubes

NUTRITION (per serving):	
Calories:	271
Fat:	Trace
% Fat calories:	Trace

Mix all ingredients in blender until creamy.

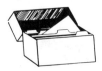

RICE CAKE CRUNCH
Prep time: 40 seconds

2 oz sliced chicken breast
5 cucumber slices
Dash of nutmeg
Dash of celery seed
1 rice cake

NUTRITION (per serving):	
Calories:	131
Fat:	2 grams
% Fat calories:	16

1. Place chicken on rice cake and add cucumber. 2. Sprinkle on spices.

STRAWBERRY YOGURT FRAPPÉ
Prep time: 57 seconds

7 frozen strawberries
1 cup nonfat strawberry yogurt
1/4 cup nonfat milk (liquid)
Dash of vanilla extract

NUTRITION (per serving):	
Calories:	234
Fat:	0 grams
% Fat calories:	0

Mix all ingredients in a blender until smooth.

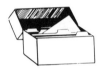

QUICK PIZZA
Prep time: 59 seconds

1 whole wheat English muffin
1 oz grated or sliced lowfat mozzarella cheese
2 tablespoons tomato sauce
1 teaspoon Italian herbs

NUTRITION (per serving):	
Calories:	210
Fat:	3 grams
% Fat calories	14

1. Spread tomato sauce on both slices of English muffin. 2. Sprinkle Italian herbs. 3. Place cheese on bread. 4. Microwave until cheese is melted.

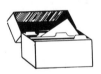

PITA PAN
Prep time: 24 seconds

1/2 large wheat pita bread
1 handful alfalfa sprouts
1 tablespoon peanut butter
1/2 banana, sliced

NUTRITION (per serving):	
Calories:	314
Fat:	9 grams
% Fat calories:	25

1. Spread peanut butter on bread. 2. Add banana. 3. Add sprouts.

FIESTA BEAN BURRITO
Prep time: 59 seconds

1/2 cup vegetarian refried beans
1 tablespoon salsa
1 teaspoon chopped cilantro (optional)
1 whole wheat tortilla

NUTRITION (per serving):	
Calories:	206
Fat:	5 grams
% Fat calories:	19

1. Spread beans over tortilla. 2. Sprinkle on remaining ingredients. 3. Heat in microwave until warm (approximately 40 seconds). 4. Roll tortilla and mixture into a burrito.

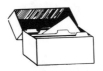

PEANUT BUTTER MELT
Prep time: 35 seconds

1 slice whole wheat bread
1/2 banana
2 teaspoons peanut butter

NUTRITION (per serving):	
Calories:	186
Fat:	7 grams
% Fat calories:	31

1. Toast bread (optional). 2. While bread is toasting, slice banana. 3. Spread peanut butter on toast and cover with banana.

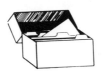

ABBA ZABBA
Prep time: 54 seconds

1 whole wheat tortilla
2 teaspoons peanut butter
2 tablespoons applesauce
1 tablespoon raisins
Dash of cinnamon

NUTRITION (per serving):	
Calories:	223
Fat:	8 grams
% Fat calories:	31

1. Warm tortilla (optional). 2. Spread remaining ingredients down the center of tortilla. 3. Roll up tortilla.

COTTAGE RAISIN TOAST
Prep time: 57 seconds

1 slice raisin bread	
1/4 cup lowfat cottage cheese	**NUTRITION** (per serving):
1 teaspoon raisins (or 1 minibox)	Calories: 119
Dash of cinnamon	Fat: 2 grams
	% Fat calories: 12

1. Toast bread. 2. Spread cottage cheese on bread. 3. Sprinkle raisins and cinnamon.

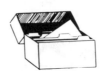

TUNA SALAD PITA
Prep time: 59 seconds

1/2 large pita pocket bread	
3-1/2 oz water-packed tuna (or one small can)	**NUTRITION** (per serving):
1/4 cup lettuce	Calories: 297
Dash of celery seed	Fat: 1 gram
Dash of pepper	% Fat calories: 4
Dash of onion powder	

1. Line pita bread with lettuce. 2. Mix spices with tuna. 3. Stuff tuna mixture into pita.

Note: You can add mayonnaise, but this will take more time and add more calories.

20

On-the-Run Eating Plan

"I know all about nutrition and diet. . . . What should I eat for dinner tonight?"—

secretary and professional dieter

Here is your nutrition Band-Aid for eating on the run: one week's worth of menus that require no cooking (except for occasionally turning on a microwave). I call this your nutrition Band-Aid because eventually you will have to plan (yes, the "p" word) and face those tricky eating situations. By now you have learned how to do this, but this one week of meals is my gift to you.

Realize that the limitation of following any set meal plan is that it can be very simple. The real challenge will be putting it together yourself. (That should be easy for you after reading this book!)

7-7-7-7 EATING PLAN

This meal plan is unique because it is flexible (to fit a variety of lifestyles and eating styles). There are seven breakfasts, seven lunches, seven snacks, and seven dinners. The meals include selections from fast food, deli menus, restaurant fare, convenience food, and, of course, one-minute meals. They are designed so that (when followed) you will get at least the 6-5-4-3-2 Nutrition Countdown servings.

Here are the basic principles that will help you meet the 6-5-4-3-2 Nutrition Countdown without cooking:

1. Any meal can be switched for another meal in the same category. For example, any lunch can be traded for any other lunch.
2. For variety's sake, try not to use more than two of the same meals in one week.
3. Although there are fast-food and convenience-food options, you are not obligated to eat them.

Meals can be broken down into smaller snacks if that helps meet your schedule. Just keep the 6-5-4-3-2 Nutrition Countdown as your guide, and you will do fine.

To assist you in following this plan, I have provided a grocery list of what you will need for the week (it's at the end of this chapter). Don't forget to stock some of the foods in your work environment, be it home, office, car, or wherever.

7 Breakfasts

I

Any fast-food chain:
Pancakes (hold the butter, easy on the syrup)
Orange juice
Nonfat or lowfat milk

II

McDonald's:
Cheerios or Wheaties
Orange juice
Lowfat milk
Apple bran muffin

III

One-minute meals:
Peach Smoothie
Cottage Raisin Toast

IV

One-minute meal:
Hula Bagel
Minibox raisins

V

One-minute meal:
English Muffin Melt
1/2 cup grape juice
1 cup lowfat milk

VI

1-2 Breakfast Bars (chapter 18)

VII

One-minute meal:
Strawberry Yogurt Frappé
1 whole wheat English muffin

7 Lunches

I

Wendy's:
Chili
Side salad
Orange juice or lowfat milk

II

Subway:
6-in. turkey breast (hold the cheese and oil;
request either vinegar or light Italian dressing
as your sandwich spread)
Veggie Salad (hold the cheese)
with light Italian dressing

III

One-minute meal:
Fiesta Bean Burrito
5 cherry tomatoes
1 graham cracker

IV

One-minute meal:
Mini-Gouda and Baguette
Vegetable juice

V

One-minute meal:
Quick Pizza
Raw zucchini slices

VI

One-minute meal:
Greek Stuffed Pita
Raw cauliflower flowerettes

VII

Coffee shop:
Garden salad or broth-based soup
(minestrone, vegetable)
Chicken breast sandwich (grilled, not fried)

7 Snacks

I

Weight Watchers microwave popcorn (or plain microwave)
2 tablespoons Parmesan cheese
Any fresh fruit

II

Nonfat fruit yogurt and 3 tablespoons Grape-Nuts
Minibox raisins

III

One-minute meal:
Cottage Cheese Delight (optional: blend with ranch dip mix)
Raw celery stalks, carrot sticks, or broccoli
2 whole wheat crackers (such as Wasa)

IV

2 Pogen Krisprolls
1 Mini-Bonbell reduced-fat cheese
15 grapes, 1 apple, or 1 orange

V

One-minute meal:
Savory Chick-Pea Spread and Pita Wedges
4 dried apricot halves

VI

1 tablespoon peanut butter and 2 rice cakes
1 banana

VII

One-minute meal:
Ak-Mak and Cheese
1 pear or kiwifruit

7 Dinners

I

Domino's Pizza:
2 slices veggie pizza (hold the olives)
Add your own:
Salad
Nonfat or lowfat milk

II

Convenience food
Any best-bet frozen meal (see Table 5.2 and Appendix A)
1 whole wheat roll
1 garden salad
1 cup nonfat or lowfat milk

III

Restaurant
Tossed salad (dressing on the side)
Fresh fish of the day, broiled without butter
1 roll
Steamed rice or potato (1-2 pats margarine)
Steamed vegetables (hold the butter)
Decaf cappuccino (request froth be made with lowfat milk)

IV

Cobbette Salad (recipe follows)
1 small French roll baguette

V

One-minute meals:
2 Tortilla Pinwheels
Peach Smoothie

VI

One-minute meal:
Submarine Cheese Melt
Carrot sticks

VII

Pasta with Tomatoes (recipe follows)
Zucchini (cook in microwave)
Garlic Cheese Bread (recipe follows)

SELECTED DINNER RECIPES

COBBETTE SALAD

2-3 cups romaine lettuce
2 tablespoons chopped chives
2 tablespoons chopped parsley
2 oz sliced turkey
1/3 cup garbanzo beans
1 slice lowfat American cheese, cut into strips
Cherry tomatoes
Fat-free dressing

Combine ingredients and toss until mixed.

PASTA WITH TOMATOES

1 package fresh angel hair pasta
1 16-oz can chopped, stewed tomatoes
Parmesan cheese
Italian herbs

1. Boil water (in microwave). Soak angel hair pasta in water for 90 seconds (or as directed). 2. Top hot pasta with stewed tomatoes, Italian herbs, and Parmesan cheese. Toss until mixed well. Microwave until hot, about 30 seconds.

GARLIC CHEESE BREAD

1 small baguette or sourdough roll
1 oz lowfat mozzarella cheese
Garlic powder

1. Place cheese on bread. 2. Top with garlic powder to taste. 3. Zap in microwave until cheese is melted.

GROCERY LIST

The purpose of this chapter has been to provide you with a week's worth of eating ideas. This should take the guesswork out of getting started and make that task much easier for you. To make the process still easier, List 20.1 is a complete grocery list for all the items you will need to eat your way through this 7-day plan.

List 20.1
Complete Grocery List for Eating Plan

This list covers all meals and snacks in this chapter. If you decide you will not opt for a certain meal or snack, make sure you delete the items from the list. Note, there will be leftovers, such as extra tortillas because they are packed in 12s!

Bread

Bagels, regular and mini size
Baguettes, 2 small
English muffin, whole wheat
Pita bread
Raisin bread
Roll, whole wheat
Tortilla, whole wheat

Canned/Packaged

Canned chick-peas/garbanzo
    beans
Crushed pineapple
Grape juice
Milk, nonfat, powdered
Peaches (packed in their own juice)
Peanut butter, natural style
Salad dressing, any fat-free
Salsa
Tomato sauce
Tomatoes, stewed, chopped
Vegetable juice
Vegetarian beans

Cereals and Crackers

Ak-mak crackers
Grape-Nuts
Pogen Krisprolls
Rice cakes
Whole grain cereal

Dairy

American cheese, sliced, lowfat
Cottage cheese, lowfat
Feta cheese
Laughing Cow, reduced cheese
    cubes
Milk, lowfat or skim
Milk, powdered nonfat
Mini Bonbell reduced cheese
Mozzarella cheese, lowfat

Parmesan cheese
Ricotta cheese, lowfat
Swiss cheese, lowfat
Yogurt (nonfat):
    1 vanilla
    1 strawberry
    3 any fruit flavor

Deli Section

Angel hair pasta (9-oz pkg)
Turkey, sliced

Frozen

Boysenberries
Strawberries (fresh is best, if in
    season)
Any best bet frozen dinner (See
    Appendix A)

Produce

Apple
Banana
Berries
Broccoli
Carrots
Cauliflower
Celery
Cherry tomatoes
Chives (scallions)
Cilantro (like parsley)
Dried apricot halves
Garlic (fresh)
Kiwifruit
Lettuce—1 head romaine, 1 head
    green leaf
Melon
Minibox of raisins
Pear
Spinach
Tomato
Zucchini

Spices

Cinnamon
Garlic powder
Italian herbs
Nutmeg
Paprika
Vanilla extract

Other

Lemon juice (fresh or bottled)
Tahini (sesame seed paste) or
    sesame seeds
Honey

21

One-Minute
Wrap-Up

"Sometimes I feel like I have to be a nutritional encyclo-
pedia to eat right."—

engineer

You are only a bite away from healthy eating. Remember, progress not perfection is what truly matters. Minor eating indiscretions will not affect your health or weight. It's the consistent pattern that counts.

Tackle only one problem area at a time and build on your successes. Even little steps can have big results. For example, consider the impact of these changes over one week (see p. 189).

It should be clear that without changing where you eat but just by modifying a little of what you eat, you can make a substantial impact, without being a diet martyr.

You would save your body from nearly 48 pounds' worth of calories over one year, if you made the above changes (which are relatively painless). You can do that!

Regardless of your lifestyle or eating habits (be it fast food or frozen cuisine), it is possible to eat nutritiously in a minimal amount of time. You *can* eat on the run and eat right.

Eating on the Run Modification

Day	Instead of	Have	Calorie savings
1	*McDonald's* McDLT	*McDonald's* Small hamburger	320
2	*Taco Bell* Taco Salad	*Taco Bell* Bean Burrito	590
3	*Stouffer's* Turkey Potpie	*Healthy Choice* Breast of Turkey	250
4	*Subway* 12-in. Tuna Sub	*Subway* 12-in. Turkey Sub	459
5	*Hardee's* Big Country Breakfast with sausage	*Hardee's* Pancakes	570
6	*Jack-in-the-Box* Ultimate Cheeseburger	*Jack-in-the-Box* Chicken Fajita Pita	650
7	*Arby's* 1 pkg Honey French salad dressing	*Arby's* Lemon wedge, or calorie-free (your own)	350
	Total savings at the end of one week:		**3,189**
	Total savings at the end of one year:		**165,828**

22

One-Minute Information

"I didn't realize how making a few changes could be so easy and yet make a difference."—
freelance photographer

This chapter provides quick and handy reference information that you may have always wanted to know but were too busy to find out. You may find a few surprises. The information was derived from sources listed in the reference section. In this chapter you will find the following:

Section 1: Foods That are Good for You

- 15 Naturally Occurring Low-Calorie Foods
- Leanest Meats
- Nutritional Power of Beans
- 21 High-Fiber Foods
- 15 High-Carbohydrate Foods

Section 2: Foods to Limit

- 15 High-in-Hidden-Fat Foods
- 15 Common High-Cholesterol Foods

- 15 High-Sodium Foods
- 15 Common Sources of Hidden Sugar
- 15 High-Calorie Beverages
- 15 Caffeine Sources

Section 3: For Further Information

- Percent Saturated Fat Content in Oils
- Toll-Free Numbers for Food Companies

SECTION 1: FOODS THAT ARE GOOD FOR YOU

---

15 Naturally Occurring Low-Calorie Foods

Food	Calories
1 tbsp chives	1
1 tbsp onions, raw, chopped	3
1/2 cup endive	4
1/2 cup lettuce	4
1/2 cup alfalfa sprouts	5
1/2 cup cabbage, raw	5-10
1 stalk celery	6
1/2 cup spinach, raw, chopped	6
10 radishes	7
1/2 cup cucumber, sliced	7
1/2 cup greens, raw (collard, dandelion, mustard, turnip)	7-13
1/2 cup parsley, chopped	10
1/2 cup eggplant	11
1/2 cup cauliflower	12
1/2 cup mung beans	13

Leanest Meats (≤ 2 g of fat per oz; data based on cooked weight)

Beef	Fat (g) per oz
Select round: Top round roast, steak	1.5
Select round: Eye round roast, steak	1.7
Choice round: Top round roast, steak	1.8
Choice round: Eye round roast, steak	1.9
Select round: Tip roast, steak	1.9
Select round: Round steak	2.0
Chicken (without skin)	
Breast	1.0
Drumstick	1.6
Egg	
Egg white	0
Fish	
Tuna (light, water-packed)	0.1
Cod, scallops, and lobster	0.2
Shrimp, crab (blue, canned), haddock, perch, pollack, pike, and whitefish	0.3
Crayfish, grouper	0.4
Crab, Alaska king, and snapper	0.5
Clams and rockfish	0.6
Tuna (white, water-packed) and sea bass	0.7
Trout and halibut	0.8
Salmon (chinook, smoked)	0.9
Mussels	1.3
Oysters	1.4
Sturgeon	1.5
Swordfish	1.5
Sole	2.0
Lamb	
Foreshank, braised	1.7
Leg shank, roasted	1.9
Pork	
Loin, tenderloin (roasted)	1.4
Turkey (without skin)	
Light meat	0.9
Turkey ham	1.2
Veal	
Cubed, lean	1.2
Shoulder (arm, blade, or whole)	1.5-1.8
Sirloin	1.8

Data adapted from California Department of Health Services, 1990.

Nutritional Power of Beans

Beans go a long way nutritionally. The following is based on a one-cup portion, cooked. Note that in most cases one cup of beans will meet your entire folic acid needs for the day!

	Calories	Protein (g)	Iron (mg)	Folic Acid (micrograms)	Fiber[a] (g)
RDA[b]	—	44-50	10-15	180-200	—
Black	227	15	4	256	12
Black-eyed peas	198	13	4	356	9
Chick-peas	269	15	5	282	8
Great Northern	210	15	4	181	10
Kidney	225	15	5	229	13
Lentils	231	18	7	358	10
Lima	217	15	5	156	8
Navy	259	16	5	255	13
Pinto	235	11	4	294	11
Split peas	231	16	3	127	5

[a]There is no RDA for fiber. Most health authorities recommend 20-35 grams of dietary fiber per day.

[b]The RDA listed is based on ages 15 and older for males or females.

Data adapted from J.W. Anderson, 1990, and Pennington, 1989.

21 High-Fiber Foods

Food	Dietary Fiber (g)[a]
1 oz whole grain cereal	4-14
1 cup beans (pinto, split pea, etc.)	5-13
1 cup frozen okra, cooked	8
1 cup frozen peas, cooked	8
1 cup frozen brussels sprouts, cooked	7
1 large pear	6
2/3 cup cooked oatmeal	5
1 cup whole wheat spaghetti	5
2 slices German rye bread	5
1 cup French-style green beans	5
1 guava	5
1/2 cup turnip, cooked	5
1/2 cup sweet potato, cooked	4
1 cup whole wheat macaroni	4
3 tablespoons wheat germ	4
3/4 cup blackberries	4
1/2 small mango	3
1 cup fresh raspberries	3
1 small orange	3
2 figs	3
1 small apple with skin	3

[a]These numbers have been rounded off.

Data adapted from J.W. Anderson, 1990.

15 High-Carbohydrate (CHO)
Foods Containing at Least 75% CHO Calories[a]

Food	CHO (g)
1 cup dried fruit (apples, apricots, currants, figs, peaches, prunes, raisins)	57-130
1 cup Grape-Nuts	94
1 exotic fruit (mango, papaya, plantain, pomelo, sapodilla, sapota)	30-76
1 roll, hoagie/submarine	75
10 dates	61
3 pancakes	57
1 cup rice	50
1 cup cereal (All-Bran, 100% Bran Flakes, Bran Buds, Cracklin' Bran, Fruit & Fibre, Raisin Bran, Wheat & Raisin Chex)	41-62
1 cup sweet potato, mashed	49
1 cup succotash	47
1 cup fruit juice/nectars	27-45
1 cup lima beans	40
1 cup corn	39
1 cup pineapple	39
1 cup noodles	39

[a]The recommended carbohydrate intake is at least 58% of daily calories and, for athletes, at least 60-70% of daily calories.

SECTION 2: FOODS TO LIMIT

15 High-in-Hidden-Fat Foods[a]

Food	% Fat calories
Olives (black, green)	99
Baking chocolate	95
Nuts, seeds (almonds, beechnuts, Brazil nuts, butternuts, cashews, filberts, hickory, macadamia, peanuts, pecans, pilinuts, walnuts; pumpkin, sesame, sunflower)	73-93
Cream cheese	91
Avocado	88
Coleslaw	80-87
Coconut (meat, milk)	79-85
Pâté	79-85
Frankfurter (beef or turkey)	83
Pork sausage and bacon	82
Sardines, in oil	81
Pepperoni	81
Kielbasa	80
Chorizo	80
Liverwurst	80

[a]The recommended fat level is no more than 30% of daily calories.

15 Common High-Cholesterol Foods

Food	Cholesterol (mg)
3 oz liver (beef, pork, or chicken)	300-536
3 oz giblets (chicken or turkey)	334-355
1 serving soufflé	240-339
1 serving quiche	113-240
1 serving flan	214
1 chicken egg	213
1 éclair	187
1 piece sponge cake	164
1 oz cod-liver oil	160
1 cup French vanilla ice cream, soft-serve	153
1 serving chocolate mousse	142
1/2 cup custard	136
3 oz shrimp	128
3 oz sardines	119
1 piece lemon meringue pie	98

15 High-Sodium Foods[a]

Food	Sodium (mg)
1 cup soup/gravy, canned or packaged	637-3,865
3 oz dried, chipped beef	3,650
1 entrée, frozen or canned	700-3,500
1 fast-food entrée	290-3,300
1 tbsp bacon bits	2,753
1 tsp salt	1,955
1 tsp onion or garlic salt	1,620-1,850
1 tsp meat tenderizer	1,750
1 oz teriyaki sauce	1,380
1 tbsp soy sauce	1,029
1 link pork sausage	1,020
1/2 cup sauce (cheese, curry, hollandaise, sour cream, stroganoff, barbecue)	503-1,109
1 medium dill pickle	928
1 cup cottage cheese	850
1 tsp baking soda	821

[a]The recommended sodium intake is a maximum of 2,400 mg/day.

15 Common Sources of Hidden Sugar

Barbecue sauce
Shake 'n Bake
Luncheon meats
Granola bars
Breakfast cereals
Catsup
French dressing
Fruit drinks
Honey
Corn syrup
Soup, canned or packaged
Spaghetti sauce, canned or packaged
Chewable vitamin/mineral supplements
Eggnog
Canned fruit, in syrup

15 High-Calorie Beverages

Beverage	Calories
8 oz coconut milk	552
10 oz milk shake	317-350
1 cup eggnog	342
1 standard beer, sweet wines, cocktails	153-335
1 cup instant breakfast with whole milk	287
1 cup Ovaltine with whole milk	227-265
12 oz fruit drinks, ades, punch	144-242
1 cup malted milk	236
1 cup hot chocolate	218
1 cup chocolate milk	208
1 cup prune juice	181
12 oz soda pop	156-178
1 cup goat milk	168
1 cup whole milk	157
1 cup grape juice	155

15 Caffeine Sources[a]

Food/Nonprescription Drug	Caffeine (mg)
Standard dose Prolamine	280
Standard dose Dexatrim, Dietac	200
Standard dose No Doz, Vivarin	100-200
6 oz automatic drip coffee	181
6 oz automatic perk coffee	125
Standard dose aspirin	30-128
6 oz hot tea (strong)	65-107
6 oz iced tea	70-75
6 oz instant coffee	54-75
12 oz cola beverages	32-65
12 oz Mountain Dew	54
12 oz Mello Yellow	51
8 oz chocolate milk	48
2 oz chocolate candy	45
1 oz baking chocolate	45

[a]The recommended caffeine intake is less than 250 mg/day.

SECTION 3: FOR FURTHER INFORMATION

Percent Saturated Fat Content in Oils

Highest	%	Lowest	%
Coconut oil	86	Canola oil	6
Palm kernel oil	81	Safflower oil	10
Butter	66	Sunflower oil	11
Palm oil	48	Corn oil	13
Beef fat (tallow)	48	Olive oil	14
Pork fat (lard)	40	Soybean oil	15
Chicken fat	32	Peanut oil	18
Vegetable shortening	28	Margarine	19
Cottonseed oil	26		

Saturated fat in the diet should not exceed 10% of your total daily calories.

Toll-Free Numbers for Food Companies

Here's a fast method of asking a question or sending a quick comment to a food company without writing a letter: toll-free numbers.

Arby's	800/ 2-ADVISE
Betty Crocker	800/ 328-6787
Burger King	800/ YES-1800
Campbell Soup Company	800/ 257-8443
Dial Corporation (Lunch Buckets, Armour)	800/ 528-0849
Domino's Pizza	800/ DOMINOS
Formagg	800/ 441-9419
General Foods Corporation	800/ 431-1003
General Mills	800/ 231-0308
Kibun Products International	800/ 542-8626
Kraft	800/ 323-0763
Healthy Choice	800/ 323-9980
Hormel	800/ 523-4635
Laura Scudder's	800/ 426-7336
Lawry's Foods	800/ 952-9797
Mrs. Field's Cookies	800/ 344-2447
Nabisco Brands	800/ 932-7800
Pillsbury	800/ 767-4466
Procter & Gamble	800/ 543-7276
Ragú	800/ 243-5804
Sara Lee	800/ 323-7117
Subway	800/ 888-4848
Togo's	800/ 698-6467
Tyson Foods	800/233-6332

Related Hotline Numbers

American Dietetic Association	800/ 877-1600
Bulimia Anorexia Self Help	800/ 227-4785
Cancer Information Service	800/ 4-CANCER
National Health Information Center	800/ 336-4797
USDA Meat and Poultry Hotline	800/ 535-4555

Appendix A

Frozen Foods: "Light" Meals Nutritional Data

Information compiled from manufacturers' data. Items marked with an asterisk (*) are considered Best Bets. These items have no more than 30% fat calories and no more than 800 mg of sodium.

Entrée	Calories	Fat (g)	% Fat calories	Sodium (mg)	Cholesterol (mg)
Armour Classics Lite					
Baby Bay Shrimp	220	6	25	890	105
Beef Pepper Steak	220	4	16	970	35
*Beef Stroganoff	250	6	22	510	55
*Chicken ala King	290	7	22	630	55
*Chicken Burgundy	210	2	9	780	45
Chicken Marsala	250	7	25	930	80
*Chicken Oriental	180	1	5	660	35
Salisbury Steak	300	11	33	980	40
Seafood with Natural Herbs	190	2	9	1,020	35

(Cont.)

Entrée	Calories	Fat (g)	% Fat calories	Sodium (mg)	Cholesterol (mg)
Armour Classics Lite (Continued)					
Shrimp Creole	260	2	7	900	45
*Steak Diane	290	9	28	440	80
Sweet and Sour Chicken	240	2	8	820	35
Budget Gourmet Light Dinners					
Breast of Chicken	250	5	18	830	40
Roast Chicken	270	9	30	1,010	55
Sirloin of Beef	260	10	35	680	60
Sliced Turkey Breast	290	8	25	1,050	45
*Teriyaki Chicken	290	9	28	780	35
Budget Gourmet Light Entrées					
Beef Stroganoff	290	12	37	570	85
*Cheese Lasagna with Vegetables	290	9	28	780	15
Cheese Ravioli	290	10	31	930	55
Chicken Au Gratin	250	11	40	870	50
Chicken Enchilada Suiza	290	12	37	810	40
French Recipe Chicken	240	9	23	1,000	50
*Glazed Turkey	270	5	17	760	40
Ham and Asparagus Au Gratin	290	12	37	1,170	50
Lasagna with Meat Sauce	300	13	39	760	40
Linguini with Scallops and Clams	290	11	34	710	45
*Mandarin Chicken	300	7	21	670	40
*Orange Glazed Chicken	250	3	11	350	10
Oriental Beef	290	9	19	810	30
Sirloin Beef in Herb Sauce	270	10	33	720	60
Sirloin Enchilada Ranchero	280	10	32	750	15
Sirloin Salisbury Steak	260	13	45	700	65
Dining Lite					
Beef Teriyaki	270	5	17	850	45
*Cheese Cannelloni	310	9	26	650	70
*Cheese Lasagna	260	6	21	800	30
*Chicken ala King	240	7	26	780	40
*Chicken Chow Mein	180	2	10	650	30
*Chicken with Noodles	240	7	26	570	50
Fettuccine with Broccoli	290	12	37	1,020	35
*Glazed Chicken	220	4	16	680	45
*Lasagna with Meat Sauce	240	5	19	800	25
Oriental Pepper Steak	260	6	21	1,050	40
Salisbury Steak	200	8	36	1,000	55
Spaghetti with Beef	220	8	33	440	20
Sauce and Swedish Meatballs	280	10	32	660	55

Entrée	Calories	Fat (g)	% Fat calories	Sodium (mg)	Cholesterol (mg)
Healthy Choice Dinners					
*Beef Pepper Steak	290	6	17	530	65
*Breast of Turkey	290	5	16	420	45
*Chicken and Pasta Divan	310	4	12	510	60
*Chicken Oriental	220	2	8	460	55
*Chicken Parmigiana	280	3	10	310	60
*Herb Roasted Chicken	260	3	10	300	40
*Mesquite Chicken	310	2	6	270	45
*Salisbury Steak	300	7	21	480	50
*Shrimp Creole	210	1	4	560	65
*Shrimp Marinara	220	1	4	320	50
*Sirloin Tips	290	6	19	350	70
*Sole Au Gratin	270	5	17	470	55
*Sweet and Sour Chicken	280	2	6	260	50
*Yankee Pot Roast	260	4	14	310	45
Kraft Eating Right					
Beef Pepper Steak	290	10	31	400	35
*Beef Sirloin Tips and Noodles	250	8	29	340	70
*Chicken Breast Parmesan	300	10	30	540	50
*Chicken Breast and Vegetables	200	4	18	570	30
*Fettucini Alfredo	220	7	29	410	20
*Glazed Chicken Breast	240	4	15	560	35
*Lasagna with Meat Sauce	270	7	23	440	30
*Macaroni and Cheese	270	8	27	590	15
*Shrimp Vegetable Stir Fry	150	4	24	400	50
Sirloin Salisbury Steak	230	8	31	510	50
*Sliced Turkey Breast	250	7	25	560	50
*Swedish Meatballs	290	7	22	470	55
Lean Cuisine					
*Baked Cheese Ravioli	240	8	30	590	55
Beef and Bean Enchanadas	280	10	32	890	60
Beef and Pork Cannelloni	260	10	35	950	45
Beefsteak Ranchero	270	9	30	950	40
*Breast of Chicken Marsala	190	5	24	400	80
Breast of Chicken Parmesan	260	8	27	870	80
Breast of Chicken with Herb Cream Sauce	260	10	35	910	80
*Broccoli and Cheddar Toppped Potato	290	9	28	590	55
Cheese Cannelloni with Tomato Sauce	260	10	35	910	35

(Cont.)

Entrée	Calories	Fat (g)	% Fat calories	Sodium (mg)	Cholesterol (mg)
Lean Cuisine (Continued)					
*Cheese Pizza (French Bread)	310	10	29	750	15
*Chicken à l'Orange	260	5	17	430	55
Chicken and Vegetables with Vermicelli	270	8	27	980	45
Chicken Cacciatore	250	7	25	860	45
Chicken Chow Mein	250	5	18	980	35
Chicken Enchilada	270	9	30	850	65
*Chicken in Barbeque Sauce	260	6	21	500	50
*Chicken Italiano	290	8	25	490	45
*Chicken Oriental	230	6	23	790	100
*Chicken Tenderloins in Peanut Sauce	290	7	22	530	45
Fiesta Chicken	250	6	22	880	45
*Filet of Fish Divan	260	7	24	750	85
Filet of Fish Florentine	230	8	31	840	110
Filet of Fish Jardiniere with Soufléed Potatoes	290	10	31	840	110
Glazed Chicken	270	8	27	810	55
*Homestyle Turkey	230	5	20	550	50
Lasagna with Meat Sauce	270	8	27	970	60
Linguini with Clam Sauce	270	7	23	890	30
*Macaroni and Beef	240	6	23	590	40
*Macaroni and Cheese	290	9	28	550	30
Meatball Stew	250	10	36	940	85
Oriental Beef	250	7	25	900	45
Rigatoni Bake	260	10	35	870	40
Salisbury Steak	280	15	48	840	100
Shrimp and Chicken Cantonese	270	9	30	920	100
*Sliced Turkey Breast in Mushroom Sauce	240	7	26	790	50
Spaghetti with Beef and Mushrooms	280	7	22	940	25
*Spaghetti with Meatballs	280	7	23	490	35
Stuffed Cabbage	220	10	41	930	55
*Swedish Meatballs	290	8	25	590	50
Szechuan Beef	260	10	35	680	100
Tuna Lasagna	270	10	33	890	35
Turkey Dijon	270	10	33	900	60
Vegetable and Pasta Mornay	280	11	35	970	35
Zucchini Lasagna	260	7	24	950	25
LeMenu Healthy Dinners					
*Cheese Tortellini	230	6	23	460	15
*Glazed Chicken	230	3	12	480	55

Entrée	Calories	Fat (g)	% Fat calories	Sodium (mg)	Cholesterol (mg)
*Herb-Roasted Chicken	240	7	26	400	70
*Salisbury Steak	280	9	29	400	35
*Sliced Turkey	210	5	21	540	30
*Stuffed Shells	280	8	26	690	25
*Sweet and Sour Chicken	250	7	25	530	40
*Turkey Divan	260	7	24	420	60
*Veal Marsala	230	3	12	700	75

Ultra Slim Fast

Entrée	Calories	Fat (g)	% Fat calories	Sodium (mg)	Cholesterol (mg)
*Beef Pepper Steak and Parsleyed Rice	270	4	14	690	45
Chicken and Vegetables	290	3	10	850	30
Chicken Fettuccine	380	12	29	980	65
Country Style Vegetable and Beef Tips	230	5	21	960	45
*Mesquite Chicken	360	1	3	300	65
*Pasta Primavera	340	9	24	730	25
Roasted Chicken in Mushroom Sauce	280	6	20	830	55
*Shrimp Creole	240	4	15	730	80
Shrimp Marinara	290	3	10	880	70
Spaghetti with Beef and Mushroom Sauce	370	10	25	990	25
*Sweet and Sour Chicken	330	2	6	340	45
Turkey Medallions in Herb Sauce	280	6	20	950	40

Weight Watchers

Entrée	Calories	Fat (g)	% Fat calories	Sodium (mg)	Cholesterol (mg)
*Angel Hair Pasta	210	5	21	420	20
*Baked Cheese Ravioli	290	9	28	630	85
Beef Enchiladas Ranchero	230	10	39	720	40
*Beef Fajitas	250	7	25	630	20
Beef Salisbury Steak Romana	190	7	33	470	40
*Beef Sirloin Tips and Mushrooms in Wine Sauce	220	7	29	540	50
*Beef Stroganoff	290	9	28	600	25
*Broccoli and Cheese Baked Potato	290	8	25	600	25
Cheese Enchiladas Ranchero	360	18	45	900	60
*Cheese Manicotti	280	8	26	490	75
*Cheese Pizza	300	7	21	630	35
*Cheese Tortellini	310	6	17	570	15
*Chicken ala King	240	6	23	490	20
Chicken Burrito	310	13	38	790	60
Chicken Cordon Blue	220	9	37	630	50

(Cont.)

Entrée	Calories	Fat (g)	% Fat calories	Sodium (mg)	Cholesterol (mg)
Weight Watchers (Continued)					
*Chicken Divan Baked Potato	280	4	13	730	40
Chicken Enchiladas Suiza	280	11	35	600	30
*Chicken Fajitas	230	5	20	590	30
*Chicken Fettuccine	280	9	29	590	40
Chicken Kiev	230	9	35	610	30
Chicken Nuggets	270	12	40	540	50
*Deluxe Combination Pizza	330	10	27	650	25
Deluxe French Bread Pizza	330	12	33	800	30
Fettucini Alfredo	210	8	34	600	35
*Fillet of Fish Au Gratin	200	6	27	700	60
*Garden Lasagna	290	7	22	670	20
*Ham Lorraine Baked Potato	250	4	14	670	15
*Homestyle Chicken and Noodles	240	7	26	450	30
*Homestyle Turkey Baked Potato	300	6	18	670	60
*Imperial Chicken	240	3	11	640	35
Italian Cheese Lasagna	350	12	31	690	30
*Lasagna with Meat Sauce	320	10	28	630	45
*London Broil in Mushroom Sauce	140	3	19	510	40
*Oven Fried Fish	240	7	26	380	15
Pasta Primavera	260	11	38	800	5
*Pasta Rigati	300	9	27	490	25
Pepperoni French Bread Pizza	320	11	31	830	30
*Pepperoni Pizza	320	10	28	710	35
*Sausage Pizza	320	10	28	630	35
Southern Fried Chicken	320	16	45	690	65
*Spaghetti with Meat Sauce	280	7	23	610	25
Stuffed Turkey Breast	260	10	35	910	80
*Sweet 'n Sour Chicken Tenders	240	1	4	600	40
*Veal Patty Parmigiana	190	6	28	650	55

Appendix B

Fast Food Nutritional Data

Fast Food	Calories	Fat (g)	% Fat calories	Sodium (mg)	Cholesterol (mg)
Arby's					
Breakfast					
Biscuit					
Bacon	330	19	52	960	10
Ham	325	17	47	1,190	30
Plain	280	15	48	730	0
Sausage	460	32	62	1,000	60
Cinnamon Nut Danish	340	10	25	230	0
Croissant					
Bacon and Egg	469	25	47	580	280
Ham and Cheese	345	20	53	960	100
Mushroom and Cheese	337	18	47	625	98
Plain	260	16	54	300	49
Sausage and Egg	600	38	56	619	406

(Cont.)

Fast Food	Calories	Fat (g)	% Fat calories	Sodium (mg)	Cholesterol (mg)
Arby's					
Breakfast (Continued)					
Platter					
Ham	719	24	30	1,192	404
Sausage	816	39	43	841	428
Toastix	420	25	54	440	20
Desserts					
Apple Turnover	303	18	50	178	0
Cherry Turnover	280	18	57	200	0
Chocolate Chip Cookie	130	4	28	95	0
Salads					
Chef	210	11	47	720	115
Chicken Cashew	590	37	56	1,140	65
Garden	149	9	52	99	74
Side	25	0	0	30	0
Salad Dressings					
Blue Cheese	390	39	90	766	28
Honey French	350	27	69	532	0
Light Italian	25	1	36	255	0
Thousand Island	345	33	77	576	13
Sandwiches					
Bac'n Cheddar Deluxe	526	37	62	1,672	83
Beef 'n Cheddar	455	27	53	955	63
Chicken Breast Sandwich	493	25	46	1,019	91
Chicken Cordon Bleu	630	37	52	1,824	138
Corned Beef Sandwich	400	15	34	1,440	45
Fish Fillet Sandwich	537	29	49	994	79
Ham 'n Cheese	292	14	42	1,350	45
Philly Beef 'n Swiss	460	28	56	1,300	107
Reuben	450	18	36	1,900	55
Roast Beef					
Giant Roast Beef	531	23	39	908	65
Junior Roast Beef	218	9	35	345	20
King Roast Beef	467	19	37	766	49
Regular	353	15	38	588	39
Super	501	22	40	798	40
Steak Deluxe	800	51	57	460	65
Steak 'n Cheddar	640	37	52	960	45
Sub Deluxe	540	29	48	1,600	50
Turkey Deluxe	375	17	40	1,047	39
Shakes					
Chocolate	451	12	23	341	36
Jamocha	368	11	25	262	35
Vanilla	330	12	31	281	32

Fast Food	Calories	Fat (g)	% Fat calories	Sodium (mg)	Cholesterol (mg)
Side Orders					
Cheddar Fries	399	22	49	454	9
Curly Fries	337	17	46	167	0
French Fries	246	13	48	114	0

Burger King

	Calories	Fat (g)	% Fat calories	Sodium (mg)	Cholesterol (mg)
Breakfast					
Bagel	272	6	20	438	29
Bagel with Cream Cheese	370	16	39	523	58
Bagel Sandwich with:					
Bacon, Egg, and Cheese	453	20	40	872	252
Egg and Cheese	407	16	35	759	247
Ham, Egg, and Cheese	438	17	35	1,114	266
Sausage, Egg, and Cheese	626	36	52	1,137	293
Biscuit	332	17	46	754	2
Biscuit with:					
Bacon	378	20	48	867	8
Bacon and Egg	467	27	52	1,033	213
Sausage	478	29	55	1,007	33
Sausage and Egg	568	36	57	1,172	238
Croissant	180	10	50	285	4
Croissan'wich with:					
Bacon, Egg, and Cheese	361	24	60	719	227
Egg and Cheese	315	20	57	607	222
Ham, Egg, and Cheese	346	21	55	962	241
Sausage, Egg, and Cheese	534	40	67	985	268
Danish (Typical)	500	36	65	288	6
French Toast Sticks	538	32	54	537	80
Hash Browns	213	12	51	318	3
Scrambled Egg Platter	549	34	56	893	365
Scrambled Egg Platter with Bacon	610	39	58	1,043	373
Scrambled Egg Platter with Sausage	768	53	62	1,271	412
Burgers					
Cheeseburgers					
Bacon Double	515	31	54	748	105
Bacon, Double, Deluxe	592	39	59	804	111
Barbecue Bacon Double	536	31	52	795	105

(Cont.)

Fast Food	Calories	Fat (g)	% Fat calories	Sodium (mg)	Cholesterol (mg)
Burger King					
Burgers (Continued)					
Deluxe	390	23	53	652	56
Double Deluxe	483	27	50	851	100
Mushroom Swiss Double	473	27	51	746	95
Regular	318	15	42	661	50
Hamburger					
Deluxe	344	19	50	496	43
Regular	272	11	36	505	37
Whopper					
Regular	614	36	53	865	90
with Cheese	706	44	56	1,177	115
Double	844	53	57	933	169
Double with Cheese	935	61	59	1,245	194
Dessert					
Apple Pie	311	14	41	412	4
Salads					
Chef	178	9	46	568	103
Chunky Chicken	142	4	25	443	49
Garden	95	5	47	125	15
Side	25	0	0	25	0
Salad Dressings					
Bleu Cheese	300	32	96	512	58
French	290	22	68	400	0
Olive Oil and Vinegar	310	33	96	214	0
Ranch	350	37	95	316	20
Reduced Calorie Light Italian	170	18	95	762	0
Thousand Island	290	26	81	403	36
Sandwiches and Nuggets					
Bk Broiler Chicken Sandwich	379	18	43	764	53
Chicken Sandwich	685	40	53	1,417	82
Chicken Tenders	236	13	50	541	46
Fish Tenders	267	16	54	870	28
Ocean Catch Fish Filet	495	25	45	879	57
Shakes					
Chocolate	326	10	28	198	31
Chocolate with Syrup Added	409	11	24	248	33
Strawberry with Syrup Added	394	10	23	230	33
Vanilla	334	10	27	213	33

Fast Food	Calories	Fat (g)	% Fat calories	Sodium (mg)	Cholesterol (mg)
Side Orders					
French Fries	341	20	53	241	21
(medium, salted)					
Onion Rings	302	17	51	559	3

Carl's Jr.

Breakfast					
Bacon (2 strips)	45	4	80	150	5
Breakfast Burrito	430	26	54	740	285
Cinnamon Rolls	460	18	35	230	0
Danish (all varieties)	520	16	28	230	0
English Muffin with Margarine	190	5	24	280	0
French Toast Dips	490	26	48	60	40
Hash Brown Nuggets	270	17	57	410	5
Hot Cakes with Margarine	510	24	42	1,190	15
Sausage (1 patty)	190	18	85	520	30
Scrambled Eggs	120	9	68	105	245
Sunrise Sandwich	300	13	39	550	160
Sunrise Sandwich with Bacon	370	19	46	750	120
Sunrise Sandwich with Sausage	500	32	58	990	165
Burgers					
Cheeseburgers					
Classic Double	710	47	60	1,050	110
Double Western Bacon	1,030	63	55	1,810	145
Hamburgers					
Famous Star	610	38	56	890	50
Happy Star	320	14	39	590	35
Old Time Star	460	20	39	810	50
Super Star	820	53	58	1,120	105
Western Bacon	730	39	48	1,490	90
Desserts					
Blueberry Muffin	340	9	24	300	45
Bran Muffin	310	7	20	370	60
Chocolate Cake	380	20	47	335	70
Chocolate Chip Cookie	330	17	46	170	5
Fudge Brownie	430	19	40	210	trace
Miscellaneous					
Jr. Crisp Burrito (each)	140	7	45	200	65
Shakes (regular size)	350	7	18	230	15

(Cont.)

Fast Food	Calories	Fat (g)	% Fat calories	Sodium (mg)	Cholesterol (mg)
Carl's Jr. (Continued)					
Potatoes					
Bacon and Cheese	730	43	53	1,670	45
Broccoli and Cheese	590	31	47	830	25
Cheese	690	36	49	1,160	40
Fiesta	720	38	48	1,470	15
Lite	290	1	3	60	0
Sour Cream and Chive	470	9	36	180	20
Salads					
Chicken Salad-To-Go	200	8	36	300	70
Garden Salad-To-Go (large)	100	5	45	410	10
Garden Salad-To-Go (small)	50	3	54	75	5
Taco Salad-To-Go	310	19	55	920	75
Salad Dressings (1 oz)					
Blue Cheese	150	15	90	250	20
House	110	11	90	170	10
Italian	120	13	98	210	0
Reduced Calorie French	40	2	45	290	0
Thousand Island	110	11	90	200	5
Sandwiches					
Charbroiler BBQ Chicken Sandwich	400	7	15	880	40
Charbroiler Chicken Club Sandwich	570	29	46	1,160	60
Country Fried Steak Sandwich	720	43	54	1,420	50
Filet of Fish Sandwich	550	26	43	940	90
Roast Beef Club Sandwich	620	34	49	1,950	45
Roast Beef Deluxe Sandwich	540	26	43	1,340	40
Side Orders					
French Fries (regular)	420	20	43	200	0
Onion Rings	520	26	45	960	0
Zucchini	390	23	53	1,040	0
Dairy Queen Brazier					
Burgers					
Cheeseburger					
Single	410	20	44	790	50

Fast Food	Calories	Fat (g)	% Fat calories	Sodium (mg)	Cholesterol (mg)
Double	650	37	51	980	95
Triple	820	50	55	1,010	145
Hamburger					
Single	360	16	40	630	45
Double	530	28	48	660	85
Triple	710	45	57	690	135
Hot Dogs					
DQ Hounder	480	36	68	1,800	80
with Cheese	533	40	68	1,210	89
with Chili	575	41	65	1,900	89
Hot Dog					
Regular	280	16	51	830	45
with Cheese	330	21	57	990	55
with Chili	320	20	56	985	55
Super Hot Dog	520	27	47	1,365	80
with Cheese	580	34	53	1,605	100
with Chili	570	32	51	1,595	100
Sandwiches and Nuggets					
All White Chicken Nuggets	276	18	59	505	39
Chicken Sandwich	670	41	55	870	75
Chicken Breast Fillet	608	34	56	725	78
Chicken Breast Fillet with Cheese	661	38	52	921	87
Fish Fillet	430	18	37	674	40
Fish Fillet with Cheese	483	22	41	870	49
Fish Sandwich	400	17	38	875	50
Fish Sandwich with Cheese	440	21	43	1,035	60
Side Orders					
French Fries	200	10	45	115	10
French Fries (large)	320	16	45	185	15
Onion Rings	280	16	51	140	15
Domino's Pizza					
2 Slices of Large (16-in. Pie)					
Cheese	376	10	24	483	19
Deluxe	498	20	37	954	40
Double Cheese and Pepperoni	545	25	42	1,042	48
Ham	417	11	24	805	26

(Cont.)

Fast Food	Calories	Fat (g)	% Fat calories	Sodium (mg)	Cholesterol (mg)
Domino's Pizza					
2 Slices of Large (Continued)					
(16-in. Pie)					
Pepperoni	460	18	34	825	28
Sausage and Mushroom	430	16	33	552	28
Veggie	498	19	33	1,035	37
El Pollo Loco					
Chicken					
Charbroiled Chicken Salad	200	4	16	375	65
Chicken (2 pieces)	310	18	51	460	n/a
Chicken Sandwich	290	7	20	375	65
Combo Meal (2 pieces Chicken, Salsa, Corn, Coleslaw, and 3 Corn Tortillas)	720	28	33	890	n/a
Side Orders					
Beans	110	1	12	450	n/a
Coleslaw	80	6	67	160	n/a
Corn	110	2	14	110	n/a
Dole Whip	90	0	0	18	n/a
Potato Salad	140	8	50	500	n/a
Rice	100	1	9	250	n/a
Salsa	10	0	0	90	n/a
Tortillas, Corn (3)	210	2	8	70	n/a
Tortillas, Flour (3)	280	7	22	450	n/a
Hardee's					
Breakfast					
Big Country Breakfast:					
Bacon	660	40	55	1,540	305
Country Ham	670	38	51	2,870	345
Ham	620	33	48	1,780	325
Sausage	850	57	60	1,980	340
Biscuit 'N' Gravy	440	24	49	1,250	15
Biscuit Sandwiches:					
Bacon	360	21	53	950	10
Bacon and Egg	410	24	53	990	155
Bacon, Egg, and Cheese	460	28	55	1,220	165
Canadian Rise 'N' Shine	470	27	52	1,550	180
Chicken	430	32	52	1,370	45

Fast Food	Calories	Fat (g)	% Fat calories	Sodium (mg)	Cholesterol (mg)
Country Ham	350	18	46	1,270	170
Country Ham and Egg	400	22	50	1,600	175
Ham	320	16	45	1,000	15
Ham and Egg	370	19	46	1,050	160
Ham, Egg, and Cheese	420	23	49	1,270	170
Rise 'N' Shine	320	18	51	740	0
Sausage	440	28	57	1,100	25
Sausage and Egg	490	31	57	1,150	170
Steak	500	29	52	1,320	30
Steak and Egg	550	32	52	1,370	175
Cinnamon 'N' Raisin Biscuit	320	17	48	510	0
Hash Rounds	230	14	55	560	0
Pancakes (3)	280	2	6	890	15
Pancakes (3) with Bacon	350	9	23	1,110	25
Pancakes (3) with Sausage	430	16	33	1,290	40
Syrup	120	trace	0	25	0
Burgers					
Bacon Cheeseburger	610	39	58	1,030	80
Big Deluxe Burger	500	30	54	760	70
Big Twin	450	25	50	580	55
Cheeseburger	320	14	39	710	20
Hamburger	270	10	33	490	20
Mushroom 'N' Swiss Burger	490	27	50	940	70
Quarter-Pound Cheeseburger	500	29	52	1,060	70
Dessert					
Apple Turnover	270	12	40	250	8
Big Cookie	250	13	47	240	5
Cool Twist Cone (all)	190-200	6	27-28	65-100	15-20
Cool Twist Sundae					
Caramel	330	10	27	290	20
Hot Fudge	320	12	34	270	25
Strawberry	260	8	28	115	15
Salads					
Chef	240	15	56	930	115
Chicken N' Pasta	230	3	12	380	55
Garden	210	14	60	270	105
Side	20	trace	0	15	0
Sandwiches and Stix					
All Beef Hot Dog	300	17	51	710	25

(Cont.)

Fast Food	Calories	Fat (g)	% Fat calories	Sodium (mg)	Cholesterol (mg)
Hardee's					
Sandwiches and Stix (Continued)					
Chicken Fillet	370	13	32	1,060	55
Chicken Stix					
6 pieces	210	9	39	680	35
9 pieces	310	14	41	1,020	55
Fisherman's Fillet	500	24	43	1,030	70
Grilled Chicken	310	9	26	890	60
Sandwich					
Hot Ham 'N' Cheese	330	12	33	1,420	65
Roast Beef					
Regular	260	9	31	730	35
Big	300	11	33	880	45
Turkey Club	390	16	37	1,280	70
Shakes					
Chocolate	460	8	16	340	45
Strawberry	440	8	16	300	40
Vanilla	400	9	20	320	50
Side Orders					
French Fries (regular)	230	11	43	85	0
French Fries (large)	360	17	43	135	0
French Fries (big)	500	23	41	180	0
Crispy Curls	300	16	48	840	0
Jack in the Box					
Breakfast					
Breakfast Jack	307	13	38	871	203
Hash Browns	156	11	63	312	0
Pancake Platter	612	22	32	888	99
Pancake Syrup	121	0	0	3	0
Sausage Cresent	584	43	66	1,012	187
Scrambled Egg Platter	559	32	51	1,060	378
Scrambled Egg Pocket	431	21	44	1,060	354
Supreme Cresent	547	40	66	1,053	178
Burgers					
Bacon Cheeseburger	705	45	57	1,127	85
Cheeseburger	315	14	40	746	41
Double Cheeseburger	467	27	52	842	72
Grilled Sourdough	712	50	63	1,140	109
Burger					
Hamburger	267	11	37	556	26
Jumbo Jack	584	34	52	733	73
Jumbo Jack with Cheese	677	40	53	1,090	102
Ultimate Cheeseburger	942	69	66	1,176	127

Fast Food	Calories	Fat (g)	% Fat calories	Sodium (mg)	Cholesterol (mg)
Desserts					
Cheesecake	309	18	51	208	63
Double Fudge Cake	288	9	28	259	20
Hot Apple Turnover	348	19	49	316	<1
Salads					
Chef	325	18	50	900	142
Mexican Chicken	442	23	47	1,500	89
Side	51	3	53	84	<1
Taco	503	31	55	1,600	92
Salad Dressings					
Bleu Cheese	262	22	76	918	18
Buttermilk House	362	36	90	694	21
Reduced-calorie French	176	8	41	600	0
Thousand Island	312	30	87	700	23
Sandwiches and					
* Other Entrées*					
Beef Fajita Pita	333	14	38	635	45
Chicken Fajita Pita	292	8	25	703	34
Chicken Strips (4)	285	13	41	695	52
Chicken Strips (6)	451	20	40	1,100	82
Chicken Supreme	641	39	55	1,470	85
Egg Rolls (3)	437	24	48	957	29
Egg Rolls (5)	753	41	49	1,640	49
Fish Supreme	510	27	48	1,040	55
Grilled Chicken Fillet	408	17	38	1,130	64
Ham and Turkey Melt	592	36	55	1,120	79
Sirloin Cheesesteak	621	30	43	1,450	79
Taco	184	11	53	414	18
Taco, Super	281	17	54	718	29
Taquitos (5)	362	15	37	462	24
Taquitos (7)	511	21	37	681	34
Shakes					
Chocolate	330	7	19	270	25
Strawberry	320	7	20	240	25
Vanilla	320	6	17	230	25
Side Orders					
French Fries (small)	219	11	45	121	0
French Fries (regular)	351	17	44	194	0
French Fries (jumbo)	396	19	43	219	0
Onion Rings	380	23	54	451	0
Tortilla Chips	139	6	39	134	<1

(Cont.)

Fast Food	Calories	Fat (g)	% Fat calories	Sodium (mg)	Cholesterol (mg)
Kentucky Fried Chicken					
Chicken Pieces					
Extra Tasty Crispy					
Center Breast	342	20	53	790	114
Drumstick	204	14	62	324	71
Side Breast	343	22	58	748	81
Thigh	406	30	67	688	129
Wing	254	19	67	422	67
Lite 'N Crispy					
Center Breast	220	12	49	416	57
Drumstick	121	7	52	196	51
Side Breast	204	12	55	417	53
Thigh	246	17	61	386	80
Original Recipe					
Center Breast	283	15	48	672	93
Drumstick	146	9	55	275	67
Side Breast	267	17	57	735	77
Thigh	294	20	61	619	123
Wing	178	12	61	372	64
Sandwiches and Nuggets					
Chicken Littles Sandwich	169	10	53	331	17
Colonel's Chicken Sandwich	482	27	50	1,060	47
Kentucky Nuggets (6)	276	17	55	840	71
Kentucky Nuggets (9)	414	26	57	1,260	107
Side Orders					
Buttermilk Biscuit	235	12	46	655	1
Coleslaw	119	7	53	197	5
Corn-on-the-Cob	176	3	15	21	1
French Fries	244	12	44	139	<2
Mashed Potatoes and Gravy	71	2	25	339	1
Long John Silver's					
Baked Entrées					
Baked Chicken	140	4	26	670	70
Baked Fish	120	1	8	120	110
Baked Fish with Lemon Breadcrumb Sprinkle	160	2	15	440	95
Baked Fish with Scampi Sauce	180	6	30	340	90
Baked Shrimp Scampi	120	5	38	610	205

Fast Food	Calories	Fat (g)	% Fat calories	Sodium (mg)	Cholesterol (mg)
Desserts					
Lemon Meringue Pie	260	7	24	270	<5
Pecan Pie	510	25	44	470	70
Dinners					
Chicken Plank Dinner—3 pieces (3 Chicken Planks, Fryes, Slaw, 2 Hushpuppies)	830	39	42	1,340	55
Chicken Plank Dinner—4 pieces (4 Chicken Planks, Fryes, Slaw, 2 Hushpuppies)	940	44	42	1,660	70
Battered Shrimp Dinner (6 piece)	740	37	45	1,100	90
Battered Shrimp Dinner (9 piece)	860	45	47	1,470	125
Breaded Shrimp Feast (13 piece)	880	41	42	1,320	90
Breaded Shrimp Feast (21 piece)	1,070	51	43	1,790	80
Catfish Fillet Dinner	860	42	44	990	65
Clam Dinner	980	45	41	1,200	15
Fish and Chicken	870	40	41	1,520	70
Fish and Fryes—2 piece	660	30	41	1,120	60
Fish and Fryes—3 piece	810	38	42	1,630	85
Fish and More	800	37	42	1,390	70
Fish Dinner (3 piece)	960	44	41	1,890	100
Homestyle Fish Dinner (3 piece)	880	42	43	980	75
Homestyle Fish Dinner (4 piece)	1,010	50	45	1,180	90
Homestyle Fish Dinner (6 piece)	1,260	64	46	1,590	130
Homestyle Fish Sandwich Platter	870	38	39	1,110	55
Seafood Platter	970	46	43	1,540	70
Shrimp and Fish Dinner	770	37	43	1,250	80
Shrimp, Fish, and Chicken Dinner	840	40	43	1,450	80
Salads					
Coleslaw	140	6	39	260	15
Garden	170	9	48	380	<5
Ocean Chef	250	9	32	1,340	80

(Cont.)

Fast Food	Calories	Fat (g)	% Fat calories	Sodium (mg)	Cholesterol (mg)
Long John Silver's					
Salads (Continued)					
Seafood	270	7	23	670	90
Side	20	trace	0	20	0
Salad Dressings					
Bleu Cheese	120	2	15	380	<5
Malt Vinegar	2	<1	0	20	0
Ranch	140	3	19	350	<5
Reduced Calorie Italian	18	1	50	670	<5
Sea Salad	140	7	45	260	<5
Side Orders					
Breaded Clams	240	12	45	410	<5
Breaded Shrimp	190	10	47	470	40
Clam Chowder with Cod	140	6	39	590	20
Corn-on-the-Cob with Whirl	270	14	47	95	<5
Fryes	220	10	41	60	<5
Green Beans	30	trace	0	540	<5
Gumbo with Cod and Shrimp Bobs	120	8	60	740	25
Homestyle Fish Sandwich	510	22	39	780	45
Hushpuppy (1)	70	2	26	25	<5
Mixed Vegetables	60	2	30	330	0
Rice Pilaf	250	3	11	660	0
McDonald's					
Breakfast					
Apple Bran Muffin	190	0	0	230	0
Biscuit with:					
Bacon, Egg, and Cheese	440	26	54	1,230	275
Sausage	440	29	59	1,080	49
Sausage and Egg	520	35	60	1,250	275
Spread	260	13	44	730	1
Cereals					
Cheerios	80	1	11	210	0
Wheaties	90	trace	0	220	0
Danish					
Apple	390	18	41	370	25
Cinnamon Raisin	440	21	43	430	34
Iced Cheese	390	22	50	420	47
Raspberry	410	16	35	310	26
English Muffin with Butter	170	5	26	270	9

Fast Food	Calories	Fat (g)	% Fat calories	Sodium (mg)	Cholesterol (mg)
Hashbrown Potatoes	130	7	51	330	9
Hotcakes with Butter and Syrup	410	9	20	640	21
McMuffin					
Egg	290	11	35	740	226
Sausage	370	27	53	830	64
Sausage and Egg	440	27	55	980	263
Pork Sausage	180	16	82	350	48
Scrambled Eggs	140	10	63	290	399
Burgers					
Big Mac	560	35	52	950	103
Cheeseburger	310	14	40	750	53
Hamburger	260	10	33	500	37
McDLT	580	37	57	990	109
McLean Deluxe	320	10	28	670	60
McLean Deluxe with Cheese	370	14	34	890	75
Quarter Pounder	410	21	45	660	86
Quarter Pounder with Cheese	520	29	51	1,150	118
Dessert					
Apple Pie	260	15	51	240	6
Chocolaty Chip Cookies	330	16	43	280	4
McDonaldland Cookies	290	9	29	300	0
Vanilla Cone (frozen yogurt)	100	1	5	95	5
Yogurt Sundaes					
Hot Caramel	270	3	9	180	13
Hot Fudge	240	3	12	170	6
Strawberry	210	1	5	95	5
Salads					
Chef	230	13	51	490	128
Chunky Chicken	140	3	19	230	78
Garden	110	7	57	160	83
Side	60	3	45	85	41
Salad Dressings					
Blue Cheese	350	35	89	750	30
Lite Vinaigrette	60	2	30	300	0
Peppercorn	400	44	98	425	35
Ranch	330	34	94	520	20
Red French Reduced Calorie	160	8	43	440	0
Thousand Island	390	38	87	500	40

(Cont.)

Fast Food	Calories	Fat (g)	% Fat calories	Sodium (mg)	Cholesterol (mg)
McDonald's (Continued)					
Sandwiches and Nuggets					
Chicken McNuggets (6)	270	15	51	580	56
Filet-O-Fish	440	26	53	1,030	50
McChicken	490	29	53	780	43
Shakes					
Chocolate	320	2	5	240	10
Strawberry	320	1	4	170	10
Vanilla	290	1	5	95	5
Side Orders					
French Fries (small)	220	12	49	110	0
French Fries (medium)	320	17	48	150	0
French Fries (large)	400	22	50	200	0
Pizza Hut					
Hand-tossed (2 slices of a medium pie)					
Cheese	518	20	35	1,276	55
Pepperoni	500	23	41	1,267	50
Super Supreme	556	25	40	1,648	54
Supreme	540	26	43	1,470	55
Pan (2 slices of a medium pie)					
Cheese	492	18	33	949	34
Pepperoni	540	22	37	1,127	42
Super Supreme	563	26	42	1,447	55
Supreme	589	30	46	1,363	48
Personal Pan (whole pizza)					
Pepperoni	675	29	39	1,225	53
Supreme	647	28	39	1,313	49
Thin 'n Crispy (2 slices of medium pie)					
Cheese	398	17	38	867	33
Pepperoni	413	20	44	986	46
Super Supreme	463	21	41	1,336	56
Supreme	459	22	43	1,328	42
Taco Bell					
Burritos					
Bean Burrito with Red Sauce	447	14	28	1,148	9
Beef Burrito	493	21	38	1,311	57

Fast Food	Calories	Fat (g)	% Fat calories	Sodium (mg)	Cholesterol (mg)
Burrito Supreme	503	22	39	1,181	33
Combination Burrito	407	16	35	1,136	33
Specialty Items					
Chilito	383	18	42	893	47
Cinnamon Twists	171	8	42	234	0
Enchirito with Red Sauce	382	20	47	1,243	54
Mexican Pizza	575	37	58	1,031	52
MexiMelt	266	15	51	689	38
Nachos	346	18	47	399	9
Nachos Bell Grande	649	35	49	997	36
Nachos Supreme	367	27	66	471	18
Pintos 'N Cheese with Red Sauce	190	9	43	642	16
Taco Salad	905	61	61	910	80
Taco Salad without Shell	484	31	58	680	80
Tacos and Tostadas					
Chicken Soft Taco	210	10	43	590	44
Soft Taco	225	12	48	554	32
Soft Taco Supreme	272	16	53	554	32
Steak Soft Taco	218	11	45	456	14
Taco	183	11	54	276	32
Taco Bell Grande	335	23	62	472	56
Taco Supreme	230	15	59	276	32
Tostada with Red Sauce	243	11	41	596	16
Wendy's					
Burgers					
Big Classic	570	33	53	1,075	90
Big Classic with Cheese	640	38	53	1,370	100
Jr. Bacon Cheeseburger	430	25	52	835	50
Jr. Cheeseburger	310	13	38	770	45
Jr. Hamburger	260	9	31	570	34
Jr. Swiss Deluxe	360	18	45	765	40
Kid's Meal Cheeseburger	300	13	39	770	35
Kid's Meal Hamburger	260	9	31	570	35
Single with Everything	420	21	45	890	70
Single, plain	340	15	40	500	65
Desserts					
Chocolate Chip Cookies	275	13	43	256	15
Frosty Dairy Dessert (small)	400	14	32	220	50
Potatoes, Baked					
Bacon and Cheese	520	18	36	1,460	20

(Cont.)

Fast Food	Calories	Fat (g)	% Fat calories	Sodium (mg)	Cholesterol (mg)
Wendy's					
Potatoes, Baked (Continued)					
Broccoli and Cheese	400	16	36	455	trace
Cheese	420	15	40	310	10
Chili and Cheese	500	18	39	630	25
Plain	270	trace	0	20	0
Sour Cream and Chive	500	23	47	135	25
Sandwiches, Chili, and Nuggets					
Chicken Club Sandwich	506	25	44	930	70
Chicken Sandwich	430	19	40	705	60
Chili (regular)	220	7	29	750	45
Crispy Chicken Nuggets (6)	280	20	64	600	50
Fish Fillet Sandwich	460	25	49	780	55
Grilled Chicken Sandwich	340	13	34	815	60
Salads, Prepared					
Chef	180	9	45	140	120
Garden	102	5	44	110	0
Taco	660	37	50	1,110	35
Salad Dressings					
French	252	22	77	641	0
Hidden Valley Ranch	180	22			
Thousand Island	252	25	90	378	54
Side Orders					
French Fries (small)	240	12	45	145	0
SuperBar					
Alfredo Sauce (2 oz)	35	1	26	300	trace
Cheese Tortellini	60	trace	<1	280	5
Fettuccini Noodles (2 oz)	190	3	14	3	10
Flour Tortilla	110	3	25	220	n/a
Garlic Toast	70	3	39	65	trace
Pasta Medley (2 oz)	60	2	30	5	trace
Refried Beans (2 oz)	70	3	39	215	trace
Rotini Noodles (2 oz)	90	2	20	trace	trace
Spaghetti Meat Sauce (2 oz)	60	2	30	315	10
Spaghetti Sauce (2 oz)	30	trace	<1	345	trace
Spanish Rice (2 oz)	70	1	13	440	trace
Taco Chips (2 oz)	260	10	35	20	n/a
Taco Meat (2 oz)	110	7	57	300	25
Taco Shell	50	2	36	trace	n/a

References

American Dietetic Association. (1986). *Sports nutrition: A guide for professionals working with active people*. Chicago: Author.

American Dietetic Association. (1987). *Alphabet soup: Nutrients from food and supplements*. Chicago: Author.

American Dietetic Association. (1989). *Traveling lite*. Chicago: Author.

Anderson, J.W. (1990). *Plant fiber in foods* (2nd ed.). Lexington, KY: HCF Nutrition Research Foundation.

Anderson, S.L. (1990). A look at the Japanese dietary guidelines. *Journal of the American Dietetic Association, 90*(11), 1527-1528.

Aronson, V. (1986). Protein and miscellaneous ergogenic aids. *Physician and Sportsmedicine, 14*(5), 199.

Beer drinking and the risk of rectal cancer. (1984). *Nutrition Reviews, 42*(7), 244.

Bell, L.S., Tiglio, L.N., & Fairchild, M.M. (1985). Dietary strategies in the treatment of reactive hypoglycemia. *Journal of the American Dietetic Association, 85*(9), 1141.

Brownell, K. (1988, January). Yo-yo dieting. *Psychology Today*, p. 20.

Calabrese, A.N. (1985). *Trends à la carte*. Camden, NJ: Campbell Food Service.

California Department of Health Services. (1990). *The California daily food guide: Dietary guidance for Californians, a technical report for professionals*.

Clark, N. (1990). *Nancy Clark's sports nutrition guidebook*. Champaign, IL: Leisure Press.

Coleman, E. (1988). *Eating for Endurance*. Palo Alto, CA: Bull.

Costill, D.L. (1988). Carbohydrates for exercise: Dietary demands for optimal performance. *International Journal of Sports Medicine, 9*, 5.

Coyle, E.F. (1988). Carbohydrates and athletic performance. *Sports Science Exchange, 1*(7).

Fatis, M., Weiner, A., Hawkins, J., & VanDorsten, B. (1989). Following up on a commercial weight loss program: Do the pounds stay off after your picture has been in the paper? *Journal of the American Dietetic Association, 89*(4), 547.

Hazards of therapeutic doses of nicotinic acid. (1990). *Nutrition and the MD*, **16**(4), 1.

Jacobson, B.H. (1990). Effect of amino acids on growth hormone release. *Physician and Sportsmedicine*, **18**(1), 63.

Jenkins, D.J.A., et al. (1990). Nibbling versus gorging: Metabolic advantages of increased meal frequency. *New England Journal of Medicine*, **321**(14), 929-934.

Kanarek, R.B., & Swinney, D. (1990). Effects of food snacks on cognitive performance in male college students. *Appetite*, **14**(1), 15-27.

Layman, D.K. (1987). Do athletes need more protein? *Physician and Sportsmedicine*, **15**(2), 181.

Levine, A.S., Tallman, J.R., Grace, M.K., Purkee, S.A., Billington, C.J., & Levitt, M.D. (1989). Effect of breakfast cereals on short-term food intake. *American Journal of Clinical Nutrition*, **50**(6), 1303-1307.

Marshall, C.M. (1983). *Help or harm? Vitamins and minerals*. Philadelphia: Stickley.

McCarthy, P. (1989). How much protein do athletes really need? *Physician and Sportsmedicine*, **17**(5), 170.

Morgan, K.J. (1982). The role of snacking in the American diet. *Contemporary Nutrition*, **17**(9), 1.

Morris, B. (1988, March 15). Are square meals headed for extinction? *The Wall Street Journal*, p. 1.

Murray, R. (1987). The effects of carbohydrate ingestion on gastric emptying and fluid absorption during and following exercise. *Sports Medicine*, **4**, 322.

National Research Council. (1989). *Recommended dietary allowances* (10th ed.). Washington, DC: National Academy of Sciences.

National Research Council. (1989). *The diet and health report*. Washington, DC: National Academy of Sciences.

Pennington, J.A.T. (1989). *Bowes & Church's food values of portions commonly used* (15th ed.). Philadelphia: Lippincott.

Roth, G. (1984). *Breaking free from compulsive eating* (p. 37). New York: Bobbs-Merrill.

Seligmann, J. (1990, November 26). A lighter than airline load. *Newsweek*, p. 70.

Sherman, W. (1983). Carbohydrates, muscle glycogen, and muscle glycogen supercompensation. In M.H. Williams (Ed.), *Ergogenic aids in sport* (p. 13). Champaign, IL: Human Kinetics.

Slavin, J. (1988). Amino acid supplements: Beneficial or risky? *Physician and Sportsmedicine*, **16**(3), 221.

Staff. (1987, November). Obesity among children: It's growing bigger. *Tufts University Diet & Nutrition Letter*, p. 7.

Staff. (1989, January). Overcoming the 10-pound obsession. *Tufts University Diet & Nutrition Letter*, p. 3.

Staff. (1990, June). Who's making dinner when mom or dad isn't? *Tufts University Diet & Nutrition Newsletter*, p. 7.

Studies: Bicarbonate doping has no benefits (1987). *Physician and Sportsmedicine*, **15**(12), 51.

Stunkard, A.J., & Berthold, H.C. (1985). What is behavior therapy? A very short description of behavior weight control. *American Journal of Clinical Nutrition*, **41**(4), 821.

Sweet, C.A. (1989, November). Rethinking eating out. *FDA Consumer*, pp. 6-13.

Tribole, E. (1989, August 28). Controlling cholesterol in children. *Star-News*, Pasadena, CA, p. C-5.

U.S. Department of Agriculture. (1989, July 10). *Snacks and desserts: The graze craze.* USDA news feature. Washington, DC: Author.

U.S. Department of Agriculture. (1989). Eating better when eating out. (U.S. Home and Bulletin No. 232-11). Washington, DC: Author.

U.S. Department of Agriculture. (1990). A very low boron intake. *Food & Nutrition Research Briefs.* Jan.-March, p. 1. Washington, DC: Author.

U.S. Department of Health and Human Services. (1988). *Surgeon General's Report on Nutrition and Health.* Washington, DC: U.S. Government Printing Office.

Van Horn, L., & Frank, G. (1989). Children and high cholesterol: Prevention and intervention. *Journal of the American Dietetic Association*, **89**(9), 1241.

Warshaw, H. (1990). *The Restaurant companion.* Chicago: Surrey Books.

Webb, D. (1990). *International cuisines calorie counter.* New York: M. Evans & Co.

Weinberg, L. (1989). Weight loss centers offering private label foods are growing. *Environmental Nutrition*, **12**(10), 1.

Weinstein, B. (1990). Frozen breakfast entrées: Convenience at a cost. *Environmental Nutrition*, **13**(4), 4-5.

Yetiv, J.Z. (1988). *Popular nutrition practices.* New York: Dell.

Index

About the Author

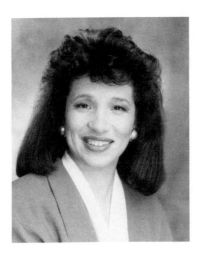

Evelyn Tribole, MS, RD, is a consulting nutritionist and freelance writer. Her column "Recipe Makeovers" appears monthly in *Shape* magazine, a national fitness publication for women. Her nutrition articles have also appeared in the *Los Angeles Times, First, Consumers Digest, Weight Watchers, Working Mother*, and the *Los Angeles Times* syndicate.

Evelyn is a national spokesperson for the American Dietetic Association and appears frequently in the national media helping consumers understand how to eat nutritiously. She conducts nutrition workshops nationwide, teaching busy people how to combine hectic lifestyles with healthy eating.

Evelyn qualified in the marathon event for the 1984 Olympic trials and was selected Young Dietitian of the Year in 1985. Evelyn recently served as the resident nutritionist for Columbia Pictures Entertainment. She holds both BS and MS degrees in nutrition from California State University–Long Beach. Evelyn lives with her husband, Jeff, and daughter, Krystin, in Irvine, California.